Hospitals and Borders

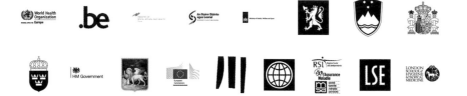

The European Observatory on Health Systems and Policies supports and promotes evidence-based health policy-making through comprehensive and rigorous analysis of health systems in Europe. It brings together a wide range of policy-makers, academics and practitioners to analyse trends in health reform, drawing on experience from across Europe to illuminate policy issues.

The Observatory is a partnership that includes the Governments of Austria, Belgium, Finland, Ireland, the Netherlands, Norway, Slovenia, Spain, Sweden and the United Kingdom; the Veneto Region of Italy; the French National Union of Health Insurance Funds (UNCAM); the World Health Organization; the European Commission; the European Investment Bank; the World Bank; the London School of Economics and Political Science (LSE); and the London School of Hygiene & Tropical Medicine (LSHTM).

Hospitals and Borders

Seven case studies on cross-border collaboration and health system interactions

Edited by

Irene A. Glinos and Matthias Wismar

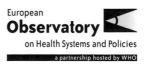

Keywords:

CASE STUDIES
DELIVERY OF HEALTH CARE
HEALTH CARE SYSTEMS
HEALTH POLICY
HOSPITALS
INTERNATIONAL COOPERATION

ISBN 978 92 890 0053 6

Printed in the United Kingdom by Bell & Bain Ltd, Glasgow

Cover design by M2M

Contents

Acknowledgements

The editors would like to express gratitude to the case study authors for their excellent work, dedication and enthusiasm during both the research and writing phases of this study: without their contributions and continued commitment the book would not have been possible. We would also like to thank our external reviewer, Pascal Garel, for incisive and constructive feedback on all nine chapters, and the internal reviewers, Rita Baeten and Nora Doering, for their valuable comments on Chapters 1 and 2. We are grateful to Lydia Wanstall for meticulous language editing, and to Jonathan North and Caroline White for unfailing support during the production process of the book.

The study is part of the Evaluating Care Across Borders (ECAB) research project, which ran for three years from 2010 to 2013 with co-funding from the European Union's Seventh Framework Programme (FP7/2007–2013) under grant agreement no. 242058. The project looked at a diverse range of topics related to cross-border health care to understand what issues, expectations and needs patients might have when seeking health care outside their home system. A total of 13 institutions across Europe took part in the project.

An overview of ECAB activities, partners and publications is available at www.ecabeurope.eu.

Irene A. Glinos and Matthias Wismar

List of tables, figures, boxes and maps

Tables

Figures

Boxes

Maps

List of abbreviations

CNAMTS	Caisse nationale de l'assurance maladie des travailleurs salariés (France)
CT	computerized tomography (scan)
DEH	district emergency hospital
DPHD	district public health directorate
DRG	diagnosis-related group
ECAB	Evaluating Care Across Borders
EEA	European Economic Association
EGTC	European Grouping of Territorial Cooperation
EHIC	European Health Insurance Card
ERDF	European Regional Development Fund
EU	European Union
EUH	European University Hospital
GDP	gross domestic product
GmbH	limited liability company
GP	general practitioner
MECSS	Maison d'enfants à caractère sanitaire et social (France)
MUMC+	Maastricht Universitair Medisch Centrum+ [Maastricht University Medical Centre] (the Netherlands)
NIHDI	National Institute for Health and Disability Insurance (Belgium)
OFBS	Observatoire Franco-Belge de la Santé [Franco-Belgian Health Observatory] (Belgium–France)
PET	positron emission tomography (scan)
RAD	radiation absorbed dose
SHI	social health insurance
UKA	Universitaetsklinikum Aachen [Aachen University Hospital] (Germany)
VHI	voluntary health insurance
ZOAST	zone organisée d'accès aux soins transfrontaliers [organized cross-border area for access to care] (Belgium–France)

List of contributors

Uta Augustin, Technical University of Berlin, Germany

Rita Baeten, Observatoire social européen, Belgium

Renate Burger, Gesundheitsmanagement, Austria

Reinhard Busse, European Observatory on Health Systems and Policies and Technical University of Berlin, Germany

Nora Doering, Maastricht University, the Netherlands/Karolinska Institutet, Sweden

Adriana Galan, National Institute of Public Health, Romania

Joan Gil, University of Barcelona, Spain

Irene A. Glinos, European Observatory on Health Systems and Policies, Belgium, and Maastricht University, the Netherlands

Ilmo Keskimäki, THL, National Institute for Health and Welfare, Finland

Régine Kiasuwa, Observatoire social européen, Belgium

Simo Kokko, Health authority of Northern Savo, Finland

Thomas Kostera, CEVIPOL and Institute for European Studies, Université libre de Bruxelles, Belgium

Riikka Lämsä, THL, National Institute for Health and Welfare, Finland

Hans Maarse, Maastricht University, the Netherlands

Victor Olsavszky, WHO Country Office, Romania

Dimitra Panteli, European Observatory on Health Systems and Policies and Technical University of Berlin, Germany

José Miguel Sanjuán, University of Barcelona, Spain

Cristian Vlădescu, University of Pharmacy and Medicine Victor Babes, Romania

Matthias Wismar, European Observatory on Health Systems and Policies, Belgium

Part I

Setting the scene, findings and conclusions

Chapter 1

Hospitals and borders: an introduction to cross-border collaboration

Irene A. Glinos and Matthias Wismar

Background

This volume examines why hospitals collaborate with each other and with other health care actors across borders in Europe. Cross-border hospital collaboration (Box 1.1) is not a new phenomenon but began to receive increased attention in the first decade of the 21st century in the context of European debates on patient mobility, the impact of European Union (EU) integration on national health systems and the particular situation of border regions. In this context, the role of health care providers stands out: while physically anchored in the health system that funds and regulates them, hospitals in border regions often witness or initiate cross-border movements of patients and health professionals.

Box 1.1. Definition of cross-border hospital collaboration

Cross-border hospital collaboration must involve at least one hospital engaging in collaborative activities with one or more health care actor(s) located in another country with the purpose of and resulting in transferring or exchanging health care-related services, knowledge and/or information. Cross-border collaboration usually involves the mobility of patients, health professionals and/or technology.

In 2003 a commentator observed, "[i]f cross-border cooperations between hospitals are now becoming 'an issue' at European level, they have already been a reality for long in Europe (the first cooperations were launched in the 70s)" (Harant, 2003). Hospital collaboration was elevated to the EU agenda in the aftermath of the Court of Justice of the European Union rulings on patient mobility (Palm et al., 2011). An informal meeting of health ministers in Malaga in February 2002 noted the added value of facilitating access to care in neighbouring countries for border region residents and called for a review of cross-border projects (Harant, 2003); both these points were reiterated by the high-level process of reflection on patient mobility and health care developments in the EU in its recommendations (European Commission, 2003).

The following years saw intense policy debates and negotiations on the EU's role in the field of health care (Mossialos et al., 2010), culminating in March 2011 in the adoption of Directive 2011/24/EU on the application of patients' rights in cross-border health care.[1] The Directive's central provisions concern the responsibilities of Member States with regard to cross-border health care (Chapter II) and the reimbursement of such costs (Chapter III) in order to facilitate access to safe and high-quality cross-border health care. The legal instrument, however, also aims to promote cooperation between EU countries (Article 1). Member States are called upon to "facilitate cooperation in cross-border healthcare provision at regional and local level" (Article 10.2), while the European Commission "shall encourage Member States, particularly neighbouring countries, to conclude agreements" and "to cooperate in cross-border healthcare provision in border regions" (Article 10.3). This places hospitals and their interactions across borders at the centre of attention.

It is essential to develop understanding of the role of hospitals, given that Member States have to comply with the Directive from 25 October 2013. Earlier studies mapped past and current cross-border projects involving hospitals across Europe (Bassi et al., 2001; Glinos, 2011; Glinos and Baeten, 2006; Harant, 2003; Palm et al., 2000). So-called promoting and hindering factors were also assessed with the intention of encouraging cross-border collaboration (Brand et al., 2007; Brand et al., 2008; Burger and Wieland, 2006; Euregio, 2011). This book proposes a different approach, considering the motivations and incentives behind such projects.

The remainder of this chapter outlines the objectives of the volume, its target audience, the conceptual framework and research questions that guided the study, the methodology and country coverage as well as the limitations of the research, and the structure of the book.

Objectives

The research presented in this volume builds on earlier contributions in the field of cross-border health care collaboration but takes a different perspective. Its purpose is not to advocate collaboration but to explore the reasons behind it, taking a neutral stance to better grasp its nature and potential merits. It is often

---

1   Directive 2011/24/EU of the European Parliament and of the Council of 9 March 2011 on the application of patients' rights in cross-border healthcare. *Official Journal of the European Union*, L 88:45–65 (http://eur-lex.europa.eu/LexUriServ/LexUriServ.do?uri=OJ:L:2011:088:0045:0065:EN:PDF, accessed 18 August 2013).

assumed that cross-border collaboration in health care is something desirable: the text of Directive 2011/24/EU openly encourages cooperation in health care provision in border regions, and many reports implicitly or explicitly favour it (Brand et al., 2007; Euregio, 2011; Euregio, 2012; Wagner and Schwarz, 2008). This positive bias means that few researchers have explored questions such as "Why does collaboration take place?" and "Who benefits?" in a critical, independent way. This volume aims to fill these gaps by expanding the scope of analysis and research to focus on three aspects in particular.

The first objective is to consider stakeholders and their intentions and motivations. Rather than a mapping exercise that tries to give a comprehensive overview of "all" cross-border projects, the case studies presented in this book dig into the underlying incentives, motivations and needs that drive hospital collaboration. Actors such as hospitals and insurers have their reasons for engaging (or not) in collaboration, but they also respond to health system needs, which in border region settings often concern patient access to services. It is essential to understand both the motivation and the need for collaboration to fully grasp why it takes place, who stands to benefit from it, and ultimately, whether it should be encouraged.

The second objective is to examine the means by which actors engage in cross-border collaboration. Understanding how collaboration works, the governance formulas used, the degrees of complexity involved and the resources required is a prerequisite to determining whether and how collaboration can be encouraged. The role of the EU as a potential sponsor of collaboration deserves particular attention.

The third and last objective is to assess how cross-border collaboration interacts with the context in which it takes place. Three dimensions are worth considering: the regional context (including geographical and demographic aspects, catchment areas, distances, transportation links and the local presence of health facilities); the health system context (including issues of capacity, competition, funding and remuneration mechanisms and volume criteria, as well as all the rules and norms at the core of health systems); and the political context (such as policy priorities, reforms and the interests of decision-makers and established stakeholder groups). All these factors influence the incentives and pressures involved in cross-border collaboration. To the editors' knowledge, this is the first study to focus on these qualitative and analytical aspects of cross-border collaboration involving health care actors.

Target audience

The choice of objectives (listed above) reflects an ambition to provide new evidence on a topic receiving increased attention in policy debates and circles.

The timing of this book coincides with the implementation of Directive 2011/24/EU. Presenting thorough scientific research developed and written to be relevant to decision-makers, the book is of interest to actors already engaged in or considering becoming involved in cross-border collaboration. Questions on feasibility, desirability and implementation are at the core of each chapter, and at the centre of the horizontal analysis in Chapter 2. The latter offers a series of eight observations drawn from the country evidence; policy conclusions directly linked to the Directive; and a "toolbox" of prerequisites necessary to start or maintain cross-border collaboration in health care. In addition to its deliberate policy perspective, the book is also relevant to observers and students of the intersection between the EU and health care known as "cross-border health care".

Conceptual framework

The overall aim of the research was to explore the incentives and roles of stakeholders – in particular those of hospitals – in setting up and steering cross-border collaboration, as well as the role of the EU in influencing cross-border collaboration. Four research questions guided the study.

1. How does collaboration between hospitals in different systems work in practice, and how are obstacles overcome? To provide the necessary background information, the first question looks at the operational elements of cross-border collaboration, including how it evolves over time and how collaborating partners respond to the specific circumstances they face. The contextual information serves to set the scene for the following analytical aspects of the research.

2. Who benefits from cross-border hospital collaboration? At the core of the study is an examination of the strategic thinking and underlying reasons behind collaboration. Researchers cannot easily assume or deduce the incentives (external factors) and motivations (conscious drivers) of partners and other stakeholders; nor will actors necessarily admit these. Thus, identifying and investigating the beneficiaries of cross-border collaboration can reveal actors' motivations and allow a more complete picture of why the collaboration takes place.

3. What role does the EU play? While many collaboration projects brand themselves as "European" or receive EU funding, there is little clarity on the extent to which collaboration is dependent on or related to EU integration, or whether it can take place independently of the EU. The third question therefore looks into the influence of the EU on cross-border collaboration.

4. What lessons can be learned from hospital collaboration in border regions? The final question serves to extract conclusions from the evidence gathered. In view of Article 10 of Directive 2011/24/EU, policy-makers and stakeholders need to know what implications the findings from the seven case studies might have for other border regions and other cross-border projects. Chapter 2 examines these issues in detail.

Methodology

The predominant research method used was in-depth qualitative analysis, based on stakeholder interviews, in order to capture the complex interplay of stakeholder incentives, needs, means and contexts and to provide fresh insights. As primary data would come from case studies, one of the early tasks was to identify and select the case studies to be included. Examples of hospitals collaborating across borders were first sought among the Evaluating Care Across Boarders (ECAB) partners. It became clear, however, that "pure" cases of hospital-to-hospital collaboration are extremely rare in Europe, as institutions that fund health care (health insurers, regional health authorities and/or national health authorities) play a part in collaboration where patient mobility is involved. The working definition of the study was therefore broadened to include non-hospital actors (see Box 1.1). The definition helped to ensure consistency across the case studies and their scope. The editors, in cooperation with the author teams, chose seven cross-border collaboration case studies from the following border regions:

- Austria–Germany, between hospitals in Braunau and Simbach
- Belgium–France, involving the hospital at Dinant and French health care actors
- Germany–Denmark, between the Flensburg Malteser hospital and Danish health authorities
- Finland–Norway, covering hospitals in Finnmark and Lapland
- the Netherlands–Germany, between Maastricht and Aachen University Hospitals
- Romania–Bulgaria, between hospitals in Călăraşi and Silistra
- Spain–France, between Catalan and French health care actors to build Cerdanya Hospital.

The mix of case studies ensures rich variety. While certain cases are well-known high-profile examples of cross-border collaboration, others have never been the subject of research, and none has been analysed in depth in the international literature. The choice of case studies also ensures sufficient diversity in both geographical coverage and nature of the collaboration, without pretending comprehensiveness. It provides a good starting point for analysing in-depth motivations, means and contexts of cross-border hospital collaborations. Geographically, evidence is drawn from Nordic and Mediterranean as well as eastern, central and western European countries. This ensures territorial as well as "political" coverage: one country is not part of the EU (Norway); two countries joined the EU in 2007 (Bulgaria and Romania); four are among the founding EU members (Belgium, France, Germany and the Netherlands); and in one country cross-border collaboration preceded EU membership (Austria). This range is particularly important in view of the third research question on the EU's role. In addition, the case studies cover a wide variety of institutional settings.

While border regions can be home to numerous cross-border initiatives, each case study zooms in on one case of collaboration. The focus is intentionally narrow to bring out the details (the evolution and history of the collaboration, geographical context, health system incentives, and so on) influencing the key players and to get as complete a picture as possible of stakeholders' behaviour and motivations.

Data for all the case studies derived primarily from stakeholder interviews. This was the method chosen in response to the research objectives and to provide new insights on the topic and complement previous studies. Case study teams followed a common research guide (outlined above) but each team was responsible for developing questionnaires and selecting interview participants based on their local knowledge of the border region. Case study authors used their discretion on how to report interviews and whether to disclose the names of interviewees. More details on the methodology of the individual case studies are provided in Chapters 3–9.

Limitations

The initial scoping process to find suitable case studies was limited by the countries represented in the ECAB project consortium (see Acknowledgements). Nevertheless, with 11 countries involved in the project (Austria, Belgium, Estonia, Finland, Germany, Hungary, Italy, the Netherlands, Slovenia, Spain and the United Kingdom), many of which do not share borders, there was a reasonable selection of border regions to choose from. Moreover, researchers who were not part of the consortium carried out two case studies.

Each cross-border collaboration inevitably represents a very specific constellation of actors, motivations, mechanisms and contexts. Under this premise, it would have been desirable to include even more case studies, but the editors hope that this limitation will be offset by future research adopting analytical frameworks similar to the one proposed in this volume.

The case studies focus their attention on a limited number of aspects of cross-border collaboration. This selective approach intentionally leaves out other dimensions.

Structure of the book

The book is composed of nine chapters divided into two sections. Part I comprises two chapters: this introduction and Chapter 2, which presents brief summaries of the country case studies, a series of horizontal observations and policy-relevant conclusions based on the analysis of the case study findings. Part II contains the seven country chapters on cross-border hospital collaborations between Austria and Germany (Chapter 3), Belgium and France (Chapter 4), Germany and Denmark (Chapter 5), Finland and Norway (Chapter 6), the Netherlands and Germany (Chapter 7), Romania and Bulgaria (Chapter 8), and Spain and France (Chapter 9).

References

Bassi D, Denert O, Garel P, Ortiz A (2001). *An assessment of cross-border cooperation between hospitals: France – Belgium – Luxembourg – Germany – Italy – Spain – Great Britain – Switzerland.* Paris, Mission opérationelle transfrontalière (www.espaces-transfrontaliers.org/document/santeanglais.pdf, accessed 18 August 2013).

Brand H, Hollederer A, Ward G, Wolf U (2007). *Evaluation of border regions in the European Union (EUREGIO), Final Report.* Brussels, European Commission (http://ec.europa.eu/health/ph_projects/2003/action1/docs/2003_1_23_frep_en.pdf, accessed 18 August 2013).

Brand H, Hollederer A, Wolf U, Brand A (2008). Cross-border health activities in the Euregios: good practice for better health. *Health Policy*, 86(2–3):245–54.

Burger R and Wieland M (2006). *Economic and sociopolitical perspectives for health services in central Europe: healthregio report.* Vienna, Gesundheitsmanagement OEG.

Euregio (2011). *Solutions for improving health care cooperation in border regions (Euregio ii).* Maastricht, Department for International Health at Maastricht University (www.euregio2-conference.eu/info/General/Final%20Report.pdf, accessed 18 August 2013).

Euregio (2012). *Guideline for the use of health technology assessment in cross border settings: a deliverable for the project – solutions for improving health care cooperation in border regions (Euregio ii Work Package 5).* Maastricht, Maastricht University (www.euregio2-conference.eu/info/General/WP5.pdf, accessed 18 August 2013).

European Commission (2003). *Report on the application of internal market rules to health services: implementation by the Member States of the Court's jurisprudence* [Commission staff working paper]. Brussels, European

Commission (http://ec.europa.eu/internal_market/services/docs/services-dir/background/2003-report health-care_en.pdf, accessed 18 August 2013).

Glinos IA (2011). Cross-border collaboration. In: Wismar M, Palm W, Figueras J, Ernst K and Van Ginneken E, eds. *Cross-border health care in the European Union: mapping and analysing practices and policies.* Copenhagen, WHO Regional Office for Europe on behalf of the European Observatory on Health Systems and Policies (Observatory Studies Series, No. 22: 217–54; www.euro.who.int/__data/assets/pdf_file/0004/135994/e94875.pdf, accessed 18 August 2013).

Glinos IA, Baeten R (2006). *A literature review of cross-border patient mobility in the European Union.* Brussels, Observatoire social européen (www.ose.be/files/publication/health/WP12_lit_review_final.pdf, accessed 18 August 2013).

Harant P (2003). Hospital cooperation in border regions in Europe. In: *Free movement and cross-border cooperation in Europe: the role of hospitals and practical experiences in hospitals, Proceedings of the HOPE Conference and Workshop, Luxembourg, June 2003.* Luxembourg, Entente des hôpitaux luxembourgeoiś:34–7.

Mossialos E, Permanand G, Baeten R, Hervey T, eds. (2010). *Health systems governance in Europe: the role of EU law and policy.* Cambridge, Cambridge University Press (www.euro.who.int/en/who-we-are/partners/observatory/studies/health-systems-governance-in-europe-the-role-of-eu-law-and-policy, accessed 18 August 2013).

Palm W, Nickless J, Lewalle H, Coheur H (2000). *Implications of recent jurisprudence on the coordination of healthcare protection systems* [report produced for the European Commission DG Employment and Social Affairs]. Brussels, Association Internationale de la Mutualite.

Palm W, Wismar M, van Ginneken W, Busse R, Ernst K, Figueras J, eds. (2011). Towards a renewed Community framework for safe, high-quality and efficient cross-border health care within the European Union. In: Wismar M, Palm W, Figueras J, Ernst K and Van Ginneken E, eds. *Cross-border health care in the European Union: mapping and analysing practices and policies.* Copenhagen, WHO Regional Office for Europe on behalf of the European Observatory on Health Systems and Policies (Observatory Studies Series, No. 22: 23–46; www.euro.who.int/__data/assets/pdf_file/0004/135994/e94875.pdf, accessed 18 August 2013).

Wagner C, Schwarz A (2008). *TK in Europe – TK analysis of EU cross-border healthcare in 2007.* Hamburg, Techniker Krankenkasse (http://www.tk.de/centaurus/servlet/contentblob/198532/Datei/1752/TK-Europa-2008-en.pdf, accessed 18 August 2013).

Chapter 2

Hospital collaboration in border regions: observations and conclusions

Irene A. Glinos and Matthias Wismar

Introduction

The chapters in this book demonstrate the potential benefits of cross-border collaboration but also show that collaboration is not easy. Of the seven collaborations studied, one has been terminated (Chapter 3), three have been called into question (Chapters 5, 6 and 7), two are at an embryonic or transitory phase (Chapters 8 and 9) and only one appears to be working smoothly (Chapter 4). One main objective of this volume is to see what lessons can be learned from the seven case studies, not only to draw conclusions but also to advance understanding of health care collaboration in border regions more broadly. This is a timely exercise, given that Directive 2011/24/EU[1] explicitly calls for "Member States to cooperate in cross-border healthcare provision in border regions" (Article 10.3). As they implement the Directive, Member States need to consider under which circumstances cross-border collaboration is likely to work, what implications it might have for domestic health systems and health actors, and how to deal with contrasting policy objectives within a legal text that asks for more collaboration but leaves patients free to bypass collaboration structures. For the European Commission, which is mandated to encourage Member States to work together in cross-border health care (Article 10.3 of the Directive), the questions of whether and how cross-border collaboration can be promoted are equally relevant. Moreover, understanding hospital collaboration is not only important in its own right but also sheds light on other aspects of cross-border cooperation in the field of health care (outlined in Chapter IV of the Directive).

---

1   Directive 2011/24/EU of the European Parliament and of the Council of 9 March 2011 on the application of patients' rights in cross-border healthcare. *Official Journal of the European Union*, L 88:45–65 (http://eur-lex.europa.eu/LexUriServ/LexUriServ.do?uri=OJ:L:2011:088:0045:0065:EN:PDF, accessed 18 August 2013).

To provide insight into these considerations, the seven case studies were analysed and key themes extracted. This chapter presents the findings, clustered into eight horizontal observations formulated as standalone propositions on the purpose, governance, context and drivers of cross-border collaboration, as well as the role of the European Union (EU) and that of individuals. The final section of the chapter presents a series of conclusions directly linked to Directive 2011/24/EU. While the chapters included in this book all involve hospitals, this chapter intentionally formulates its observations and conclusions to be relevant for observers and policy-makers concerned with cross-border collaboration involving any type of health care actor. Before presenting these observations, the next section briefly summarizes each country case study.

Chapter highlights

The following chapter summaries serve as snapshots or reminders of when, how and why each collaboration started and developed in the seven border regions studied. The brief descriptions do not cover aspects such as the specific roles of actors, their incentives and the role of the EU; these are analysed in the observations section.

Chapter 3 looks at the border region between Austria and Germany – specifically the Austrian city of Braunau and the German city of Simbach. Less than 1 km apart, divided by the River Inn, each city has its own local hospital. In 1994, when a surgical ward in the hospital at Simbach closed for renovation, German insurers contacted the Austrian hospital and signed a contract for the referral of German trauma patients. In the two decades that followed, the collaboration intensified to cover more medical areas and new agreements, including a lease contract and co-funding of a coronary angiography unit used by the wider border region population. Over the years thousands of local patients from both sides have accessed cross-border care. The collaboration has, however, suffered since the Austrian and German regional health authorities changed their policy priorities, and in 2011 it had all but ended.

Chapter 4 presents the cross-border collaboration in the Ardennes region across the French–Belgian border. In the early 2000s maternity facilities closed on the French side, prompting the mayor of Givet, French health insurers and the regional hospital authority to look for a pragmatic alternative, leading to an agreement with the Belgian hospital in Dinant, 15 km across the border, for maternity care. This turned out to be the precursor of a much broader arrangement with the creation in 2008 of the "ZOAST Ardennes": an organized zone of access to cross-border care for the border region population. The ZOAST convention, based on EU Regulation 883/2004,[2] involves the competent French regional health authority, Belgian sickness funds and several Belgian providers, and remains in place today. Thousands of local French patients have received treatment at participating Belgian hospitals.

Chapter 5 explores the cross-border arrangements allowing Danish cancer patients to access radiotherapy at the Malteser hospital in Flensburg, Germany. In 1997 a Danish cancer patient took the initiative to seek treatment at the Malteser hospital, less than 5 km across the border. This sparked the first contact between the Danish regional health authorities and the hospital, which went on to sign an agreement for radiotherapy in 1998. Cross-border collaboration intensified for 15 years, with new agreements covering more types of treatment. Some 2000 Danish patients have received care at the Malteser hospital, saving them from travelling up to 200 km to domestic providers with longer waiting times. Despite high patient satisfaction, however, cross-border collaboration was at a crossroads in 2011, as expansion of Danish radiotherapy equipment since 2008–9 has made cross-border access less necessary from the perspective of health authorities.

Chapter 6 travels north to the Arctic Circle, where the Sami-speaking population living in Finland use Norwegian ambulatory care and hospital services. A constitutional right for Sami speakers to access health and social services in their native language, combined with a shortage of Sami-speaking health professionals, led the Finnish regional health authority to look across the border. It signed a contract for specialist care with the competent Norwegian regional health authority in 2007 and two rounds of projects have encouraged cross-border collaboration. The arrangements save patients from travelling up to 700 km within Finland and facilitate access to care in a linguistic and cultural setting with which patients are familiar. Around 80–100 local Finnish patients receive treatment in Norway every year. Continuation of the collaboration is, however, in doubt, partly due to demographic challenges and temporary project financing.

Chapter 7 tells the story of Maastricht and Aachen University Hospitals, which have collaborated across the Dutch–German border since the 1990s. This initially focused on the referral of patients in need of highly specialized care, but in 2004 the two organizations signed an agreement that marked a change in the collaboration as the focus shifted to staff exchanges, and they soon hired the first professor to work simultaneously at both hospitals. In parallel to the collaboration expanding to more medical departments, the two management boards started negotiations with the intention of building a new joint centre of excellence in cardiovascular care and creating a "European University Hospital"

---

2   Regulation (EC) No 883/2004 of the European Parliament and of the Council of 29 April 2004 on the coordination of social security systems. *Official Journal of the European Union*, L 166: 1–123 (http://eur-lex.europa.eu/LexUriServ/LexUriServ.do?uri=OJ:L:2004:166:0001:0123:en:PDF, accessed 23 August 2013).

by way of a cross-border hospital merger. After years of preparation, however, the plans were called off due to a series of obstacles, and by 2012 the Maastricht–Aachen collaboration was at a crossroads.

Chapter 8 describes the case of the Călăraşi and Silistra hospitals, located 5 km apart on the Romanian and Bulgarian banks of the River Danube. Faced with significant shortages of doctors – in particular anaesthetists – the manager of Călăraşi Hospital started to look at recruiting doctors from Silistra Hospital, which has a surplus of such specialists, and recruited the first Bulgarian anaesthetist in 2008. By late 2011 a total of five Bulgarian specialists worked at both hospitals. The doctors reduce their working hours at Silistra and commute to Călăraşi around once a week for 24-hour shifts. This arrangement ensures the delivery of services in surgery and intensive care at Călăraşi. Silistra Hospital benefits from the reduced working hours, while Bulgarian specialists remain in the health system and do not migrate further away. At this early stage there is no formal collaboration between the two hospitals.

Chapter 9 examines how the project to build a new hospital on the border between Spain and France came about. Since the 1990s French women living in the region have travelled across the border to the local hospital in Puigcerdà for maternity care. The movement prompted local and regional health actors on both sides to look for a structural approach to cross-border patient flows, and in 2002 they signed an initial agreement. Thousands of local French patients have received care at Puigcerdà over the years. In parallel, local mayors pushed for the idea of building a new health facility to serve the border region population. Following lengthy preparation, Catalonia and France agreed funding in 2007, the EU committed funding in 2009, and the "European Grouping of Territorial Cooperation – Cerdanya Hospital" was created in 2010. Building work is close to completion, and Cerdanya Hospital is expected to open its doors in 2013.

Observations on hospital collaboration in border regions

This section puts forward eight observations on the purpose, governance, context and drivers of cross-border collaboration, as well as on the role of the EU and that of individuals. Each is based on the evidence gathered in the chapters and is illustrated with country examples.

1. The purpose of cross-border collaboration: integrating foreign supply and/or demand to improve patient access or share health professionals

From the perspective of providers and purchasers, collaboration can be seen as a (geographical) expansion strategy pursued to address shortages or structural weaknesses, or to strengthen their position. When a sought-after asset is available in the neighbouring system, cross-border collaboration is a way of obtaining it. Across the seven case studies it is clear that the purpose of collaboration is to incorporate supply or demand from across the border into a domestic setting, in most cases to improve patient access to health services.

- Hospitals and doctors looking for higher volumes and income seek to integrate foreign patients into their catchment areas – the newly built Cerdanya Hospital, for example, expects to attract French patients from across the border (Chapter 9; see also Chapters 3, 4 and 7).

- Purchasers facing domestic capacity constraints seek to integrate foreign facilities, workforce or equipment into their service provision (Chapters 3, 4, 5, 6 and 9). Authorities can formally recognize hospitals across the border as part of domestic capacity – as the Flensburg Malteser hospital has been for Danish cancer patients (Chapter 5), while Dinant hospital is part of the French regional planning scheme in Champagne-Ardenne (Chapter 4) – or as referral hospitals, as in the collaboration between Simbach and Braunau hospitals (Chapter 3).

- Hospitals planning to recruit or expand services seek to integrate foreign health professionals, and occasionally foreign infrastructure, into their resources – Maastricht and Aachen University Hospitals, for example, share some high-tech equipment as well as medical personnel (Chapter 7), while Călăraşi district hospital recruits commuting Bulgarian specialists (Chapter 8).

In the sample of case studies most collaborations were triggered by patients travelling for care, whether due to the closing of facilities on one side of the border (Chapters 3, 4 and 9), long travel distances within the domestic system (Chapters 4, 5, 6, 8 and 9), waiting times (Chapter 5) and/or a lack of medical personnel (Chapters 4 and 6). Cross-border access offers an opportunity for patients to overcome such inconveniences. The prominence of "patient-driven" collaboration is in line with previous studies (Glinos and Baeten, 2006; Harant, 2003) and implies that public authorities play a key role, whether visibly or behind the scenes, as they reimburse the care received abroad. Nevertheless, when health professionals are scarce, an alternative to patient mobility can be to recruit or to share workforce across the border (Chapters 3, 7 and 8). An interesting finding is that across all seven border regions some form of patient mobility is taking place, even where cross-border arrangements focus on health professional mobility (Chapters 7 and 8).

Some shortages and structural weaknesses result directly from the geography of border regions. Every case study describes one or more forms of geographical, and in some cases demographical, disadvantage. Whether involving quasi-enclaves surrounded by other territories (Chapters 4 and 7), remote regions that are underserved (Chapters 4, 5 and 6) or scarcely populated (Chapters 4, 7 and 9), the curtailment of "natural" catchment areas by borders (Chapters 3, 4, 5, 7 and 9) or the presence of physical boundaries such as rivers (Chapters 3, 6 and 8) or mountains (Chapter 9), all chapters show how the geography of borders can significantly challenge health care delivery. It is against this backdrop that partners seek so-called "cross-border solutions".

2. The governance of cross-border collaboration (i): relational, contractual or ownership-based mechanisms

The question of how cross-border collaboration works from a practical and operational perspective has attracted attention over the years (Bassi et al., 2001; Brand et al., 2007; Glinos and Baeten, 2006; Glinos et al., 2005; Glinos et al., 2010; Harant, 2006; Legido-Quigley et al., 2012; Nebling and Schemken, 2006). Even so, few have systematized the evidence, and the array of different cross-border arrangements remains hard to compare or categorize.

The case studies allow identification of three governance mechanisms. The most widely used is the simplest form of collaboration. In the business world, when firms rely on goodwill and trust to make a partnership work they are said to use "relational" governance. This minimizes contracting costs, offers flexibility and keeps partners in check when based on mutual resource dependence (Kale and Singh, 2009; Gulati, 1995). In all seven case studies partners have at some point engaged in relational governance. This is not surprising, given that resource dependency (in terms of patients, health professionals or infrastructure) often drives the collaboration, and that it requires few adaptation costs for actors belonging to different health systems: a shared need and a handshake can be enough to begin collaboration. The downside is that relational arrangements are heavily reliant on committed individuals. At Maastricht and Aachen University Hospitals, boosts and drops in the collaboration were preceded by changes in the leadership (Chapter 7); in Cerdanya, local mayors jointly pushed the cross-border hospital project forward and took their plea to Paris (Chapter 9; see also Chapters 6 and 8). Earlier studies note how the departure of enthusiastic "militants" often means the end of collaboration (Bassi et al., 2001; Harant, 2006), a point further developed in Observation 8.

Where partners want more predictability and are ready to devote some time and effort to conclude an agreement, they can make "contractual" agreements (see also Glinos et al., 2010). By creating legally binding links, contractual governance represents a more integrated approach to collaboration: it requires more commitment in terms of resources but increases stability by defining the mutual rights and obligations (Kale and Singh, 2009). While contracts may introduce some new elements into a system – for example, as the Flensburg Malteser hospital applies Danish official tariffs (Chapter 5) and Belgian hospitals open bank accounts in France to ease payments for French insurers (Chapter 4) – they generally leave existing health system structures and institutions intact. Most contractual agreements take place between the treating hospital(s) and the purchaser(s), stipulating the details of the collaboration such as the services, treatments and geographical areas covered, as well as payment modalities for patients referred abroad. Depending on the domestic health system, purchasers are either health insurers (Chapter 3) or health authorities (Chapters 4, 5 and 9). Agreements can also be concluded directly between health authorities, as between the regions of Lapland and Finnmark (Chapter 6), or between the hospital and health authorities acting as guarantor rather than purchaser to allow patients to be treated abroad (Chapter 5).

The most complex form of collaboration is when changes in ownership and legal status are involved. "Ownership" or "equity" arrangements such as mergers and joint ventures "seal" partners' commitment by aligning interests and reducing the risk of opportunistic behaviour. Such agreements are, however, difficult to negotiate (Kale and Singh, 2009; Gulati, 1995). In a cross-border setting, the purpose of collaborating becomes to create a new entity, for example, by replacing an existing one. This represents a substantial and radical change for the health systems involved and tests the partners' commitment, as innumerable technical issues need to be resolved and vast capital and time investments are necessary. Once in place, ownership agreements offer stability because they are hard to undo. The hospital in Cerdanya is a rare example of health care actors agreeing to build and co-own a hospital serving communities on both sides of the border. The project has taken over 10 years to materialize and required tireless efforts by partners (Chapter 9). When the hospital opens it will provide a testing ground for one of the most advanced forms of cross-border collaboration, yet doubts remain as to whether the hospital will function and be managed as a cross-border facility, or whether it will simply continue to treat French patients from the border region as its predecessor, Puigcerdà Hospital, has been doing for years (Gaubert, 2013; personal communication, 26 July 2013). The attempted ownership-based plans between Maastricht and Aachen University Hospitals involving a hospital merger and a jointly owned clinic (Chapter 7) show the complexity and vulnerability of such projects.

To illustrate the variation in cross-border arrangements, Table 2.1 places a selection of agreements from the seven chapters according to the three governance modes. The table shows how governance can evolve over time and be "layered".

Cross-border arrangements alternate between governance formulas reflecting the dynamic nature of interactions, the changing needs of partners and the maturity of the collaboration. In all but one case the mode or composition of partnerships changed at least once over time (Chapters 3, 4, 5, 6, 7 and 9); hence, several cases of collaboration appear more than once in the table. Initially, for example, 12 German sickness funds had contracts with the Braunau hospital, but as cross-border activities intensified, the hospital established direct agreements with the neighbouring Simbach hospital (Chapter 3). The exception is where the collaboration is so new that governance changes have not yet had time to take place (Chapter 8). Multilayered collaboration entails that partners engage in several agreements simultaneously for different aspects of health care, using different forms of integration in parallel. Maastricht and Aachen University Hospitals use binding as well as non-binding agreements (Chapter 5); other cases also show how various agreements and approaches to collaboration coexist (Chapters 4 and 6).

Table 2.1. *Selected cross-border agreements according to relational, contractual or ownership governance modes*

Relational	Contractual	Ownership
a. Hospital-to-hospital agreement (Chapter 7)	d. Hospital-to-hospital lease agreement (Chapter 3)	h. European Grouping of Territorial Cooperation (Chapter 9)
b. Hospital–purchaser tacit agreement (Chapter 4)	e. Multipartner agreement (Chapter 4)	i. Planned spin-off and merger (Chapter 7)
c. Doctor-to-doctor collaboration (Chapter 6)	f. Regional health authority agreement (Chapter 6)	
	g. Hospital–purchaser contract (Chapters 3, 4, 5 and 9)	

3. The governance of cross-border collaboration (ii): growing integration brings growing complexity

The mechanisms of relational, contractual and ownership-based collaboration present two advantages in better understanding the governance of cross-border health care: they offer a way of systematizing the diversity of cross-border practices and represent a continuum of growing integration between collaborating partners. Integration is a result of intensifying interactions and accountability relationships that make collaboration structured, formal and binding. Partners are willing to bind themselves because they derive benefits from collaboration. But while integration can improve and order complexity, it also brings complexity as partners need to coordinate, compromise and agree to align the incentives and requirements of two different health systems. This implies that with growing integration and complexity, partners need to show greater commitment.

Fig. 2.1 shows the association between integration, complexity and commitment, including at least one collaborative arrangement from each chapter. The collaboration between Călăraşi and Silistra hospitals (x: Chapter 8) is placed at the lowest level of integration and complexity since the two hospitals have not initiated any formal contracts. One level up is the inter-hospital agreement between Maastricht and Aachen University Hospitals (a: Chapter 7), which constitutes a non-binding declaration of intentions. Next is the agreement between Lapland and Finnmark health authorities (f: Chapter 6), which is binding but less complex than the following cluster of three agreements involving a dozen partners (e: Chapter 4), entailing hospital-to-purchaser contracts (g: Chapters 3, 4, 5 and 9), and including a lease contract whereby a ward was relocated from Braunau to Simbach hospital (d: Chapter 3), which approaches an equity-based arrangement. At the highest level of integration and complexity is the Cerdanya cross-border hospital, which engages Catalan and French partners as owners and managers of the newly built facility (h: Chapter 9), and the attempted but cancelled merger and infrastructure project between Maastricht and Aachen University Hospitals (i: Chapter 7). This last appears at the top of the graph because merging pre-existing organizations and creating a spin-off may be considered more complex and requires more commitment than building a new hospital to replace an older one.

Fig. 2.1. *Association between integration, complexity and commitment*

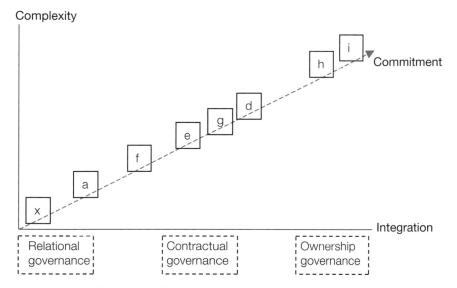

Key: letters refer to the agreements listed in Table 2.1 (see also Observation 2); x represents the early stage of collaboration between Călăraşi and Silistra hospitals (Chapter 8), which is not included in the table as no formal agreement yet exists.

Integration should be understood as a continuum where the exact starting point of relational governance remains vague (is a verbal agreement of intentions, for example, enough to consider that collaboration has started?); similarly, the highest point of integration may remain hypothetical. This book's findings and their visual representation in Fig. 2.1 lend themselves to future research: the editors intend them to develop new hypotheses and new ways of thinking about cross-border collaboration.

4. The context of cross-border collaboration (i): the need for external support

The development of cross-border collaboration depends not only on the partners directly engaged in an arrangement but also on external support, of which there are two types. Because collaboration has an impact on local supply and demand patterns, it can change the status quo of the community, the region surrounding it and the health care system involved. External actors (i.e. actors who are not part of a signed or tacit collaboration agreement) have a stake in cross-border collaboration when it affects them in some way: they can opt to support or oppose the collaboration according to whether they see their interests promoted or threatened. This can be individual actors such as local general practitioners (GPs) or providers with the power to help or to boycott cross-border collaboration by choosing to or refraining from sending patients to the collaborating hospital (Chapter 4, 7 and 9), or it can be national interests. Chapter 3 shows how private hospital and medical associations in Austria used their power to lobby lawmakers to the detriment of the collaboration, which they saw as a potential threat to salary levels. Where partners need community support, external actors must not perceive the collaboration as a means of "stealing" patients or jeopardizing the position or advantages of local actors. One way to avoid this is to provide services that complement what is available in the region and are therefore non-competitive.

In addition to community support, collaboration may need technical support in the form of financial or political sponsorship. This need usually grows as cross-border arrangements become more complex. The two examples of large-scale ownership-based projects show how the outcome of the collaboration was influenced by the ability to obtain co-funding from authorities, banks or EU programmes (Chapters 7 and 9); on the Finnish–Norwegian border, project money running out posed a risk to the continuation of collaboration (Chapter 6). Elsewhere, collaboration hinges on receiving official backing from authorities in the form of goodwill, permissions or derogations from national legislation; for example, to allow the reimbursement of care delivered abroad. The employment of Bulgarian doctors by Călăraşi Hospital is greatly facilitated by the active support of the district public health directorate and the local branch of the Romanian College of Physicians (Chapter 8; see also Chapters 3, 5, 7 and 9). Official support may also come in the form of bilateral agreements signed between authorities, such as the one between France and Belgium (Chapter 4), which provide a framework for local actors collaborating in border regions. The agreement between the French and Catalan health ministers on funding Cerdanya Hospital was an important step in a long process (Chapter 9).

Obtaining support can, however, be a lengthy and unpredictable process, swinging according to local, regional or national election results (Chapters 3, 7 and 9). Dependency on external funds and sponsors causes partners to lose a degree of control over "their" cross-border project as decision-making gravitates away from the local level and upwards in the system (Chapters 6, 7 and 9). A drawback of greater integration (see also Observation 3) can be that officialized practices may be less suited to the local environment. Local actors may be sceptical about what they see as top-down schemes of collaboration (Chapters 6 and 7). As one local actor put it, "We do not want the result of moving the [new Cerdanya] hospital one kilometre away to be that the management is hundreds of kilometres away" (Chapter 9). This point relates closely to the next observation.

5. The context of cross-border collaboration (ii): domestic health systems matter

If cross-border collaboration is to work it has to fit into the wider frameworks set by domestic health systems, which consist of institutions and incentives. Border regions are special in many ways: their demographic and geographical challenges can be acute; their proximity encourages exchanges; and they embody the places where the logic and the limits of domestic capacity planning become obvious – as a result of either a lack of services due to relative isolation (Chapters 4, 5, 6 and 9) or an abundance of services, with (university) hospitals located on each other's doorsteps (Chapters 3, 7 and 8). The combination of factors forms a context in which sharing across the border presents an advantage or an outright necessity.

Nevertheless, border regions do not escape the domestic health system of which they are part. First, institutions are domestic. Health care actors are bound by the rules, regulations and standards of the domestic health system, which cover everything from how medicine is practised and the safety and hygiene criteria to which hospitals must adhere, to how health professionals are trained and remunerated, the scope of benefit packages and how health services are paid for. This creates innumerable points of divergence between health systems and means that collaboration needs exceptions, derogations and permissions from the competent authorities when it does not play by the rules of the game. Alternatively, partners can come up with inventive solutions if they do not seek, or do not obtain, official backing.

Second, incentives are often domestic. Despite the particularities of border regions, most of the reasons stakeholders put forward in all seven chapters to explain why collaboration takes place, or not, are rooted in domestic contexts. Stakeholders first and foremost react to the incentives and constraints of the domestic scene, even when these are played out at the local, border region level, whether they involve priorities of health policies and reforms (Chapters 3, 4, 8 and 9), volume criteria (Chapters 4 and 7), remuneration mechanisms (Chapter 4), waiting time guarantees (Chapter 5), citizens' rights (Chapters 5 and 6), competitive pressures (Chapter 7) or staff shortages (Chapters 6, 7 and 8). Two chapters show how regional health authorities can shift from favouring collaboration to deterring or questioning it as domestic priorities change – in the Austrian case because collaboration did not fit new reforms for concentrating and rationalizing hospital provision (Chapter 3) and in the Danish case because new domestic capacity made collaboration less indispensable (Chapter 5).

Moreover, other factors influencing collaboration (such as the role of individuals and international competition) are also unrelated to border regions. These findings are important as they avoid any geographical determinism and go beyond "regionalistic" arguments that give disproportional attention to location aspects of collaboration. They also confirm what other research shows: that cross-border activities leave health systems, and their borders, largely intact (Kostera, 2011; 2013).

6. The drivers of cross-border collaboration: interests and needs

A key question behind the research has been to understand who benefits from cross-border collaboration (see Chapter 1). Earlier research has all too often assumed that patients benefit but rarely questioned the idea. The lesson emerging from the seven case studies is clear: patients usually benefit, but partners always benefit.

Collaboration can only work if all partners involved perceive it to be in their interests (Glinos and Baeten, 2006). While border region arrangements can benefit patients and the wider community, this is not fundamentally what drives collaboration (contrary to what stakeholders sometimes declare). This may sound simple, but in practice health care actors can be reluctant to admit the interest-driven nature of their activities, especially when seeking external funding or support for cross-border projects. Several chapters illustrate the secondary role patient preferences play. Once the priorities of the Danish regional health authorities changed, the collaboration with the Flensburg Malteser hospital needed to reinvent itself and its rationale (Chapter 5). Having begun as a solution for the purchaser (to resolve domestic undercapacity), it now represents a patient preference (thanks to shorter travel times), which may not be enough to justify its continuation. On the French–Belgian border, an extensive cross-border access zone excludes the inhabitants of one commune because the cross-border arrangement does not suit the local hospital (Chapter 4). On the German–Austrian border, the collection of tens of thousands of citizen signatures in support of the Braunau hospital did not change the Austrian regional health authorities' decision, which led to the closure of the coronary angiography unit used by both Austrian and German patients (Chapter 3).

At the same time, collaboration can only work where there is a genuine need. While patients may not drive cross-border collaboration, they vote with their feet. If patients do not perceive something (better) abroad, or if health professionals do not perceive an advantage in working across the border, cross-border collaboration has no purpose. Individuals are generally reluctant to swap their health system for something else. All case studies involving patient mobility show how cross-border arrangements are dependent on whether the local population sees a need to cross the border – usually for a type of treatment not available at proximity within the home system (Chapters 4, 5, 6, 8 and 9). Where the need is unclear, partners may struggle to define it (Chapter 7). This calls into question whether cross-border health care can be encouraged or promoted from the outside.

7. EU integration and cross-border collaboration: the many uses of the EU

Another priority for this research has been to explore the relationship between the EU and cross-border collaboration (see Chapter 1). It is often assumed that cross-border collaboration is directly and necessarily related to European integration. This may be because the EU has funded numerous projects over the years. The first "cross-border health care" projects that received support from the successive Interreg i, ii and iii programmes began in the early 1990s, and involved mainly health care actors such as hospitals and insurers (Hermans and den Exter, 1999; Harant, 2003). Later, research projects such as Europe for Patients (Rosenmöller et al., 2006), Methods of Assessing Response to Quality Improvement Strategies (Vallejo et al., 2009), and Evaluating Care Across Borders (see Acknowledgements) received funding from the EU's Framework Programmes for Research (FP6 and FP7), while projects such as Euregio i and ii (Euregio, 2008; 2011) were supported by the Public Health Programme. In parallel, the debates surrounding Directive 2011/24/EU have also contributed to putting cross-border collaboration on the agenda. Yet as the seven case study chapters of this book show, the role of the EU is far from clear.

A surprising finding has been the relatively limited role of the EU. In three case studies it did not play any active or direct role at any stage of the collaboration (Chapters 5, 6 and 8). In one additional case, collaboration started before one of the two countries involved (Austria) became a member of the EU (Chapter 3). In six cases the early phases of collaboration started as local initiatives between partners responding to a local need independently of the EU (Chapters 3, 4, 5, 6, 8 and 9). Only in the Maastricht–Aachen partnership can the origins of collaboration be traced to an EU-funded project from the early 1990s (Chapter 7).

When actors do make use of the EU, there are three main ways of doing so. First, partners use the EU to increase the legitimacy of their project when presenting it to external actors whose support they need, or when advertising the collaboration. Hospitals, for example, use Europe as a brand name when labelling their initiatives "European clinical centre" (Chapter 3), "European vascular clinic" (Chapter 7) or "European university hospital" (Chapter 7). Although the title is self-proclaimed, it can add credibility before other regional and national players. Maastricht and Aachen University Hospitals also emphasized an explicit link between their collaboration and Directive 2011/24/EU, and advertised an on-site visit by an EU health commissioner (Chapter 7). In another border region a French social health insurer added the EU flag and an Interreg logo to invoices sent to French voluntary health insurers for reimbursement of cross-border health care, despite the bills being purely a domestic matter (Chapter 4). This demonstrates use of the EU in a strategic or even manipulative way.

The EU's second role is to provide financial support. The Simbach and Braunau hospitals received €200 000 from European Structural Funds (via Interreg iiia) to improve cross-border transport of patients and medical coordination between the two hospitals (Chapter 3). The Cerdanya cross-border hospital expects to receive around €22 million through the European Regional Development Fund, representing over 50% of the total budget and making EU funding decisive for the implementation of the project (Chapter 9). On the Belgian–French border, the Observatoire Franco-Belge de la Santé (OFBS), a joint institution in receipt of Interreg funding since 1999, sets up collaboration initiatives (Chapter 4).

The third way the EU influences cross-border collaboration is through legislation. The ZOAST area of cross-border access to health care between France and Belgium is based on EU Regulation 883/2004:[3] without this

---

3   Regulation (EC) No 883/2004 on the coordination of social security systems (see *Chapter highlights* section, Note 2).

European coordination mechanism regulating the payment of care abroad, the largely successful arrangement might not have been set up (Chapter 4). Although the EU plays no active role in the Călăraşi and Silistra hospital collaboration, Romania and Bulgaria's EU membership facilitates the cross-border mobility of doctors thanks to the mutual recognition of diplomas (Chapter 8). Nevertheless, in both cases of professional mobility (Chapters 7 and 8) stakeholders perceive as cumbersome the procedure for recognizing diplomas, since medical staff cannot work at the neighbouring hospital until the formal paperwork is in order.

Finally, the EU also functions as inspiration for cross-border collaboration by creating a setting that calls into question the national logic of health care systems (Chapter 4) and makes cross-border collaboration seem a value or goal in itself. This was particularly the case in the period of "Euro-optimism" around the year 2000, ahead of enlargement and the launch of the single currency (Chapter 7).

It seems fair to say, based on the evidence gathered in this volume, that the role of the EU is ambiguous. On the one hand, several actors expressed a certain disappointment that the EU was not of greater help to their project, despite talking about cross-border collaboration (Chapters 3 and 7), and that it was too distant from local reality (Chapter 4). On the other hand, the EU legal framework and funding were indispensable for the "ZOAST" arrangement (Chapter 4) and Cerdanya Hospital (Chapter 9). Of the seven case studies, however, these two seem to be the exceptions rather than the rule.

8. The human factor in cross-border collaboration: individuals matter

Many chapters note the role of committed individuals as a key factor in collaboration; their importance extends across governance mechanisms (see also Observation 2). Several chapters show how the engagement of certain individuals, for example doctors or managers, is what allowed the collaboration to progress (Chapters 3, 6, 7, 8 and 9) and reveal that some actors made the success of a collaboration a personal project (Chapters 7 and 9). Frontrunners come to personify a project by the amount of effort they put in. Without "militants" who align their interests with cross-border collaboration and are willing to take risks – credit as well as blame – cross-border collaboration might not take off. The departure or arrival of individuals can change the game entirely. Newcomers can, for example, undo their predecessors' work if agreements or contracts have not formalized it (Chapters 6 and 7). This confirms what Bassi et al. noted on the human factor in cross-border collaboration: "individual determination and even militancy are at the origin of the most dynamic initiatives" (2001:22). It is also noteworthy how often one individual thinking "out of the box" sparked off a cross-border initiative – a patient looking for shorter waiting times (Chapter 5), a mayor in search of care within shorter distances (Chapter 4) or a hospital manager seeking extra staff (Chapter 8).

Conclusions

Building on the horizontal findings, the editors propose the following conclusions that make an explicit link to Directive 2011/24/EU. First, the evidence in this volume reveals a fundamental difference between Chapters II–III of the Directive and Chapter IV: while the former give rise to individually initiated patient mobility, the latter encourages managed mobility. According to Chapters II and III, EU citizens have the option to seek health care in another EU Member State and be reimbursed by the home state under certain conditions – for example, if the treatment is part of the national benefit package but there are delays in receiving that treatment under the national system, or if the treatment takes place in an ambulatory setting. When these conditions apply, whether or not to seek health care abroad is largely up to the individual patient. For Member States, such individually initiated patient mobility makes it hard to predict or control how many patients will exit or enter the system to seek health care. For patients, mobility under these provisions implies out-of-pocket upfront payment for medical expenses and waiting for reimbursement, which may take months; for patients with fewer means, seeking treatment abroad may therefore not be a realistic option. Cross-border collaboration, on the other hand, allows collaborating partners to set up structures to manage mobility and thus offers an alternative to Chapters II–III of the Directive. As partners can agree on the conditions for the movement of patients or professionals, cross-border flows and their implications become more predictable and influenceable for the individual as well as the system. Cross-border arrangements set up by partners save patients from having to worry about the quality of the care they receive and how to pay for it, since their usual domestic health purchaser is involved: the treating providers know which treatments patients are likely to come for and can expect swift settlement of the costs; health purchasers can decide on types of treatment and patient numbers according to the needs and requirements of their system. Moreover, cross-border collaboration allows a tailored approach: partners can share health professionals and equipment to improve service delivery and potentially save patients from having to travel. Similarly to EU Regulation 883/2004, cross-border collaboration protects patients and health systems from the risks that can be associated with cross-border care and "allows a measured approach, not hindering mobility but providing a frame in which … partners can agree on quality, volumes and prices" (Glinos et al., 2010). It is noteworthy that the best functioning collaboration out of the seven case studies is the one based precisely on Regulation 883/2004 (Chapter 4).

Nevertheless, while the chapters in this volume demonstrate the benefits collaboration can bring, they also show that cross-border collaboration is not easy. This is critical, since the Directive calls on policy-makers to facilitate and encourage collaboration. The two main reasons for the low success rate lie in the nature of cross-border collaboration – it is neither constant nor standard. First, cross-border collaboration requires a highly specific set of circumstances to work: according to the chapter findings, certain elements are necessary to initiate and develop cross-border collaboration, as summarized in Box 2.1. Collaboration is not constant because it is vulnerable to any of these factors changing. It will adapt and change according to circumstances and collapse when these are not favourable. As a general rule, health authorities prioritize domestic solutions to challenges in the health system. This reinforces the fragility of cross-border arrangements and makes their duration unpredictable. Moreover, since cross-border collaboration is context-specific, actors cannot simply transfer existing arrangements to new settings: what functions between partners in one border region may not do so in another. Second, while cross-border collaboration has its use and purpose, it should not be assumed that it is, or will become, a standard way of delivering health services. The bulk of health care will continue to be provided and consumed within national territories. The national logic underpinning health systems may show its limitations in border regions where cross-border logic is often better suited, but local and regional actors stand against the forces and interests that try to uphold the coherence of health systems. While cross-border collaboration may not be a rarity in Europe, it is still the exception rather than the rule.

For policy-makers, the burning question has to be whether and how cross-border collaboration can and should be encouraged. From a legal perspective, the European Commission receives two mandates from Article 10.3 of the Directive: to encourage Member States to conclude agreements and to encourage them to cooperate on cross-border health care provision in border regions. Both mandates, however, entail difficulties. First, convincing Member States to focus attention on cross-border care over nationally provided health care is a hard case to make. Member States may well see Commission initiatives as unwelcome EU interference in the highly complex and sensitive area of health care. For the same reason, it is unlikely that Article 10.2, which calls on Member States to facilitate cooperation, will be of great effect: they will facilitate cross-border activities where they see it as useful, independently of the Directive.

Box 2.1. *Prerequisites to initiating and maintaining cross-border collaboration in health care*

An objective, local need for cross-border collaboration: this activates and motivates partners and justifies collaboration to external actors. The need usually stems from patients who require a particular type of care locally instead of having to travel longer distances within the domestic system. It can also be that of border region hospitals seeking health professionals to fill vacant positions. If the need changes or disappears, the rationale for collaboration may do so too.

Committed individuals: collaboration is unlikely to take off without the involvement of frontrunners or "militants" who believe in the cause, push the collaboration forward and are willing to invest time and effort and take risks. If frontrunners leave, collaboration is less likely to continue.

Shared interests among partners: while partners inevitably have different and varied interests, these must not conflict. If interests clash, collaboration can quickly transform into competition. Where interests change, partners re-assess their involvement in collaboration.

Support from external actors: this can be passive, meaning that actors do not obstruct collaboration, or active. Active support usually stems from three sources: the community and stakeholders affected by cross-border collaboration (such as local doctors), public authorities that are not partners in the collaboration and funding institutions.

A suitable governance structure: this should be as simple as possible within the particularities of the border region and the purpose of the collaboration. Whether partners choose a relational, contractual or ownership-based approach to governance, it has to suit the institutions, rules and interests of the health systems involved.

Second, there is a mismatch in the locus of power. Even if the Commission is able encourage Member States, these are rarely, if ever, the initiators of cross-border collaboration. Central governments mostly take an indifferent or reluctant approach to such activities, or their position may swing according to policy agendas. The Commission has few ways to reach the local and regional actors who set up and run cross-border collaboration. Sponsoring local collaboration with EU money can have some impact but is limited by the selective nature and short duration (rarely exceeding a couple of years) of project funding. From a practical perspective, it is questionable whether cross-border collaboration can be encouraged at all: given its complexity and context-dependence, it seems not. If the prerequisites for collaboration (Box 2.1) are not in place, no amount of funding or official support can, for example, foster the need for cross-border collaboration, shared interests between partners or dedication among individuals. Where the prerequisites are in place and collaboration initiated, it is possible that external encouragement can help to cement existing practices or contribute to the funding of infrastructure. In general, policy-makers have few tools and few reasons for trying to encourage cross-border collaboration where it has not already taken root and proved its worth.

The findings echo recent studies showing that other aspects of cross-border cooperation covered by the Directive, such as recognition of prescriptions (Article 11) and reference networks (Article 12), also face considerable challenges (San Miguel et al., 2013; Palm et al., 2013). The evidence in this volume throws a new light on the utility, feasibility and desirability of cross-border collaboration, not just between hospitals but in the field of health care in general.

References

Bassi D, Denert O, Garel P, Ortiz A (2001). *An assessment of cross-border cooperation between hospitals: France – Belgium – Luxembourg – Germany – Italy – Spain – Great Britain – Switzerland.* Paris, Mission opérationelle transfrontalière (www.espaces-transfrontaliers.org/document/santeanglais.pdf, accessed 19 August 2013).

Brand H, Hollederer A, Ward G, Wolf U (2007). *Evaluation of border regions in the European Union (EUREGIO), Final Report.* Brussels, European Commission (http://ec.europa.eu/health/ph_projects/2003/action1/docs/2003_1_23_frep_en.pdf, accessed 19 August 2013).

Euregio (2008). Evaluation of cross border activities in the European Union [web site]. Düsseldorf, Landesinstitut für Gesundheit und Arbeit NRW (www.euregio.nrw.de/index.html, accessed 23 August 2013).

Euregio (2011). Solutions for improving health care cooperation in border regions [web site]. Brussels, European Hospital and Healthcare Federation (www.hope.be/06contact/contactfirstpage.html, accessed 23 August 2013).

Gaubert J (2013). *Les soins de santé transfrontaliers: approche juridique des soins médicaux transfrontaliers dans l'Union européenne* [PhD thesis]. Université Montpellier 1, 21 May.

Glinos IA, Baeten R (2006). *A literature review of cross-border patient mobility in the European Union.* Brussels, Observatoire social européen (www.ose.be/files/publication/health/WP12_lit_review_final.pdf, accessed 19 August 2013).

Glinos IA, Baeten R, Maarse H (2010). Purchasing health services abroad: practices of cross-border contracting and patient mobility in six European countries. *Health Policy*, 95(2–3): 103–12.

Glinos IA, Boffin N, Baeten R (2005). *Contracting cross-border care in Belgian hospitals: an analysis of Belgian, Dutch and English stakeholder perspectives*. Brussels, Observatoire social européen (www.ose.be/files/publication/2005/baeten_glinos_2005_BelgianCaseStudy.pdf, accessed 19 August 2013).

Gulati R (1995). Does familiarity breed trust? The implications of repeated ties for contractual choice in alliances. *Academy of Management Journal*, 38(1):85–112.

Harant P (2003). Hospital cooperation in border regions in Europe. In: *Free movement and cross-border cooperation in Europe: the role of hospitals and practical experiences in hospitals, proceedings of the HOPE Conference and Workshop, Luxembourg, June 2003*. Luxembourg, Entente des hôpitaux luxembourgeois:34–7.

Harant P (2006). Hospital cooperation across French borders. In: Rosenmöller M, McKee M, Baeten R, eds. *Patient mobility in the European Union: learning from experience*. Copenhagen, WHO Regional Office for Europe:157–77 (www.euro.who.int/__data/assets/pdf_file/0005/98420/Patient_Mobility.pdf, accessed 14 June 2013).

Hermans H, den Exter A (1999). Cross-border alliances in health care: international co-operation between health insurers and providers in the Euregio Meuse-Rhine. *Croatian Medical Journal*, 40(2):266–72.

Kale P, Singh H (2009). Managing strategic alliances: what do we know now and where do we go from here? *Academy of Management Perspectives*, 23(3):45–62.

Kostera T (2011). European dimensions of health politics in Austria: the case of cross-border healthcare [conference paper]. *2011 CPSA Annual Conference, Wilfried Laurier University Waterloo, Canada, 16–18 May*.

Kostera T (2013). Subnational responsibilities for healthcare and Austria's rejection of the EU's patients' rights directive. *Health Policy*, 111(2):149–56.

Legido-Quigley H, Glinos IA, Baeten R, McKee M, Busse R (2012). Analysing arrangements for cross-border mobility of patients in the European Union: a proposal for a framework. *Health Policy* 108(1):27–36.

Nebling T, Schemken H-W (2006). Cross-border contracting: the German experience. In: Rosenmöller M, McKee M, Baeten R, eds. *Patient mobility in the European Union: learning from experience*. Copenhagen, WHO Regional Office for Europe:137–56 (www.euro.who.int/__data/assets/pdf_file/0005/98420/Patient_Mobility.pdf, accessed 19 August 2013).

Palm W, Glinos IA, Garel P, Busse R, Rechel B, Figueras J, eds. (2013). *Building European reference networks: exploring concepts and national practices in the European Union.* Copenhagen, WHO Regional Office for Europe on behalf of the European Observatory on Health Systems and Policies (Observatory Studies Series, No. 28; www.euro.who.int/__data/assets/ pdf_file/0004/184738/e96805-final.pdf, accessed 23 August 2013).

Rosenmöller M, McKee M and Baeten R, eds. (2006). *Patient mobility in the European Union: learning from experience.* Copenhagen, WHO Regional Office for Europe (www.euro.who.int/__data/assets/pdf_file/0005/98420/ Patient_Mobility.pdf, accessed 19 August 2013).

San Miguel L, Baeten R, Remmen R, Busse R, Gil J, Knai C, Mäkinen M, Rubert G, McKee M (2013). Obstacles to the recognition of medical prescriptions issued in one EU country and presented in another. *European Journal of Public Health,* first published online 11 June 2013, doi: 10.1093/ eurpub/ckt071.

Vallejo P, Suñol R, Van Beek B, Lombarts MJ, Bruneau C, Vlcek F (2009). Volume and diagnosis: an approach to cross-border care in eight European countries. *Quality & Safety in Health Care,* 18(Suppl 1):8–14.

Part II

Border region
case studies

Chapter 3

Regional restructuring and European involvement: the ups and downs of the Braunau–Simbach hospital collaboration (Austria–Germany)

Thomas Kostera and Renate Burger

Introduction

This chapter investigates a successful hospital collaboration between Austria and Germany, in a region of Europe with close cultural and historical ties. Upper Austrian hospital KH Braunau and Bavarian hospital KKH Simbach are located on opposite sides of the River Inn, which forms the border between Austria and Germany. The collaboration began in 1994, and Austria's accession to the European Union (EU) in 1995 helped to intensify cooperation between the hospitals. The project lasted for more than a decade but was abruptly terminated at the end of 2011.

The aim of the chapter is twofold: first, to examine the Braunau–Simbach collaboration project's evolution from inception through expansion to its final form, highlighting the various phases of cooperation, the problems confronted and solutions applied; and second, to analyse the incentives and disincentives facing this type of cross-border cooperation and investigate why the project ended, despite its success. The analysis focuses on the strategies used by stakeholders to integrate incentives into the project and to manage the obstacles encountered. This approach considers not only the local and regional levels but also the national (while the German aspect is included, the focus is on Austria) and European contexts.

Both cooperating hospitals had to function within their respective national and regional political structures and their collaboration could not operate separately from these. The main argument of this chapter, therefore, is that national and regional health care reforms in the two countries had an ambivalent impact. They initially set incentives for local cross-border hospital cooperation, but the framework of the collaboration and other stakeholders' interests at the national and regional levels circumscribed the project partners' room for manoeuvre. Eventually, structural and strategic reforms decided at the regional level led to opposition to the collaboration.

Methodology

The chapter is mainly empirical in scope, using interviews and literature reviews as primary sources, as well as KH Braunau's internal magazine (*Braunauer Spitalsmagazin*) and regional newspaper articles available online. The authors conducted three hour-long interviews with the manager of KH Braunau and an official from the regional Upper Austrian Health Fund; two formed part of a doctoral research project at the Université libre de Bruxelles and one was undertaken within the framework of the Austrian "healthacross" project, a cross-border health care collaboration between Lower Austria and South Bohemia. Interviews took place in German and were translated into English by the authors, who also retrieved some data from correspondence with KH Braunau (see Annex 3.1 for interview details).

Secondary sources include literature on the Austrian welfare state, the WHO series on health systems in transition and two reports issued by the Austrian "healthacross" project, which cite the Braunau–Simbach project as an example of good practice in cross-border collaboration.

The Braunau–Simbach collaboration in operation

Context and evolution of the collaboration

The general public hospital of St Josef Braunau (KH Braunau) in Upper Austria and the district hospital at Simbach (KKH Simbach) in Bavaria are centrally located in a geographic triangle formed by Linz, Salzburg and Munich, separated by the River Inn (Map 3.1). The Franciscan nuns of Vöcklabruck run KH Braunau, set up as a limited liability company (GmbH) under Austrian law. Kreiskrankenhäuser Rottal-Inn gemeinnützige GmbH, which is a subsidiary of the Rottal-Inn district[1] in Bavaria and a non-profit-making limited liability company under German law, manages KKH Simbach (Burger and Wieland, 2010a).

Cooperation between the hospitals developed gradually and out of necessity. The "trigger" initiating the first phase of cross-border activities was a request made to the Austrian hospital by 12 Bavarian sickness funds covering the local population. The German health care system allowed sickness funds to purchase foreign ambulatory medical services. KKH Simbach underwent a restructure in 1994; this resulted in the closure of its surgical ward, and KH Braunau was asked to cooperate on emergency care because of its geographic proximity.

---

1 The district ("Landkreis") is the owner. German districts are an intermediate level of governance above municipalities and below the regional government.

Map 3.1. *Braunau–Simbach project location*

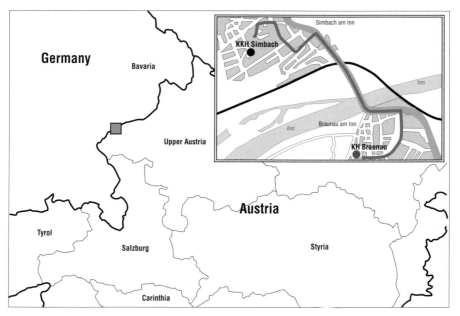

Sources: Burger and Wieland, 2010a; Wikipedia.

The sickness funds and KH Braunau created a contract that handed responsibility for an emergency care unit for trauma surgical patients to the Austrian hospital. When KKH Simbach's paediatric ward also closed in 1996, the contract was extended to cover paediatric treatment.

This cross-border service was initially provided for about 170 patients per year; the number increased to about 500 patients in 2009 (Table 3.1). The contract between KH Braunau and the Bavarian sickness funds is still valid for emergency care only (Interview 1).

Table 3.1. *German patients treated in KH Braunau (annual flows)*

Indicator	1998	2009
Total ambulant patients including cross-border commuters	1 535	2 400
Inpatients from Simbach and surroundings	240	500

Source: data provided by KH Braunau; figures on Austrian patients treated in KKH Simbach during the same period are not available.

A logical consequence of the developing cooperation process was collaboration in the activities of the regional emergency rescue dispatch centres, situated in Passau in Germany and Ried in Austria (Interview 1). KH Braunau further decided to try to extend its catchment area north of the border into

Germany, and cross-border cooperation with KKH Simbach intensified as the hospitals worked on improving the range of services available. From 1999 KH Braunau also offered computerized tomography (CT) scans for inpatients of KKH Simbach.

The second phase of cooperation began in 1999, as KH Braunau underwent a general refurbishment, which meant that wards had to close. In KKH Simbach more inpatient beds became available after a reorganization, so an internal medicine ward (capacity: 29 beds) was relocated from the Austrian to the German hospital, based on a lease contract for a period of five years. In January 2005 a second internal medicine ward (capacity: 30 beds) was relocated to KKH Simbach. Overall, KKH Simbach admitted some 1900 KH Braunau inpatients between May 2004 and July 2005. During the same period the number of German patients treated in the Austrian hospital continued to rise (Burger and Wieland, 2010a).

In August 2005 the project entered its third phase: the EU began to co-fund the Braunau–Simbach collaboration through its Interreg iiia programme, which was launched to foster intra- and extramural cross-border health care, with the aim of reducing access barriers for patients. Consequently, the German Rottal-Inn administrative district and KH Braunau initiated a process to establish a "Braunau–Simbach European clinical centre". The starting point was the need to reduce overstaffed facilities in the Austrian hospital, which lacked available space for some wards. In November 2005 KH Braunau relocated a surgical ward, setting up a surgical day care clinic in KKH Simbach, and in September 2007 the hospital owners together appointed a head of the joint German–Austrian department of internal medicine located in KKH Simbach (Burger and Wieland, 2010a). The selection procedure was based on an informal agreement, but the head of department was formally employed by both hospitals (Interview 1).

Cooperation between the hospitals continued to grow in the ensuing years. An important step in this process was the creation of a joint coronary angiography unit in July 2008, initiated by KH Braunau but located at KKH Simbach because of a lack of available space at the Austrian hospital. The service aimed to guarantee long-term cross-border care of high quality for a region with about 130 000 citizens. Investment in the facility reached €1.2 million, mainly from KH Braunau, and it provided cardiological care for both the Austrian Innviertel and the German Rottal-Inn regions. Initial calculations put projected annual patient numbers at 850, but even within the unit's first year far more examinations took place (Table 3.2).

Table 3.2. *Patients examined at the coronary angiography unit*

Indicator	2008	2010
Total examinations	2 137	2 219
Austrian patients	58.2%	60%
German patients	41.8%	40%

Sources: Interview 1; Franziskanerinnen von Vöcklabruck, 2011.

Most patients were inhabitants of the neighbouring Braunau district and Rottal-Inn region, but some came from further afield: from other Austrian provinces and regions throughout the German state of Bavaria. Before 2008 the lack of a cardiological centre meant that the local Austrian rural population had been severely underdiagnosed, and the risk of mortality after a heart attack in the region had previously been up to 30% higher than in more central parts of Austria. The new cross-border facility not only helped to reduce this disparity but also positively influenced prevention. In 2009 the Braunau–Simbach coronary angiography unit became a GmbH operated jointly by an Austrian GmbH (a subsidiary of the Franciscan nuns of Vöcklabruck) and the municipality of Simbach (with a 4.9% share). From 2009, therefore, both KH Braunau and KKH Simbach paid for additional services obtained from this newly created organization, COR GmbH (Interview 1).

Plans to expand

In 2010 the third phase of cooperation intensified in order to increase the financial stability and future development of the cross-border collaboration. Negotiations about integrating four regional hospitals (Braunau in Austria; Simbach, Eggenfelden and Pfarrkirchen in Germany) into a joint European clinical centre began. The aim was to create centres of excellence and set medical priorities to enhance the quality of care. The joint organization would offer increased efficiency, and the plan's objectives thus included not only better medical care but also significantly reduced costs.

The proposed European clinical centre would result in close cooperation between all the regional hospitals. A joint hospital organization would offer cross-border inpatient and outpatient care at four different locations for the whole region, encompassing both Rottal-Inn and Braunau. The new project aimed to ensure the sustainable preservation of all four hospital sites while saving costs. As well as primary and secondary care, the joint organization would focus on services for specific diseases (such as cardiology, traumatology and visceral surgery), with each location establishing itself as a regional centre of excellence for specific medical activities and serving as a mutual gatekeeper for the group. Overall hospital planning in both countries would integrate all services provided by the centres of both countries, with reimbursement handled according to the country-of-origin principle. Planned negotiations with health insurance companies and other utility providers, however, did not materialize (Burger and Wieland, 2010b).

Regional hospital restructuring and project termination

In 2011 an abrupt change occurred on the German side of the project. German hospital operator and collaboration partner Kreiskrankenhäuser Rottal-Inn gemeinnützige GmbH decided to pool intensive care in its three hospitals at Eggenfelden, Pfarrkirchen and Simbach in Eggenfelden (40 km from Braunau) for economic reasons. As a result, at the beginning of 2011 the internal medicine ward moved out of KKH Simbach. Following this closure, the hospital wards leased by KH Braunau at KKH Simbach also catered for German patients; this meant an increase in work for the Austrian partner to avoid a loss of patients (*Braunauer Spitalsmagazin*, March 2011). The German hospital operator also wanted to make the leased stations available to increase the number of beds in the psychosomatic ward (e-mail correspondence with KH Braunau, September 2011), as it had decided on a strategic reorientation to transform KKH Simbach into a specialist hospital for psychosomatic treatment (MeinBezirk.at, 2011).

Pressure to reorganize also increased on the Austrian side in June 2011 as the Upper Austrian regional government developed a new hospital strategy. This aimed to reduce the number of beds in various regional hospitals, simplify organizational structures and create savings of €336 million on projected hospital spending to 2020 (Land Oberösterreich, 2011a). The government ordered KH Braunau to develop a plan to repatriate the wards leased from KKH Simbach to reduce organizational costs and concentrate available hospital beds more effectively within the region (MeinBezirk.at, 2011). It also instructed the Austrian hospital to stop purchasing cardiological services from the jointly founded COR GmbH by the end of 2011 (*Braunauer Spitalsmagazin*, June 2011). This forced the closure of COR GmbH, despite KH Braunau's previous investment in the organization, and the cross-border collaboration came to an end in December 2011 (e-mail correspondence with KH Braunau, September 2011). The German partner subsequently employed a cardiologist and created a coronary angiography unit in Eggenfelden in January 2012 (Rottal-Inn Kliniken, 2012).

Problems and solutions

As the final evolution of the project shows, the main obstacles to cross-border cooperation between KH Braunau and KKH Simbach stemmed from largely national – and thus territorial – conceptions of health care provision. Structural reforms and strategic reorientations had a negative impact on the collaboration. In addition, other problems arose within the daily routines of running a bi-national hospital structure, for which the hospital managers created solutions on a case-by-case basis. The hospitals are subject to two different bodies of national legislation; treating patients of two nationalities in one hospital demands a de facto "adjustment" of the legislation, but this was not possible within the framework of the collaboration. The following practical examples that arose during the project are typical of the problems that had to be tackled. They are limited to core issues mentioned in interviews and do not represent an exhaustive list.

An initial issue arose when Austrian health officials insisted that Austrian patients be treated by Austrian health professionals and according to Austrian safety standards. This territorial argument created a disincentive related to the secondment of workers: Austrian physicians employed by an Austrian hospital are subject to Austrian social security for their own health and pension insurance, but an Austrian physician working on a ward in Germany is seconded to the other country, meaning that German legislation applies. To avoid problems with social insurance legislation, KH Braunau let physicians rotate between the hospitals to ensure that the Austrian physicians would not endanger their pension and health insurance benefits (Interview 2).

A further obstacle to the treatment of Austrian patients on a German ward involved national regulations of building standards for hospitals. Initially, the Austrian state official responsible insisted on an Austrian examination and official approval of KKH Simbach according to Austrian building regulations. Austrian technicians, however, do not have authorization to examine a hospital on German soil. A decision that Austrian authorities would ask for official administrative assistance if an Austrian patient complained about the German building eventually resolved this problem. While these considerations of building safety represent a virtual rather than a tangible obstacle to the daily routine, the issue of national responsibility for the safety of buildings was one that had to be tackled (Interview 1).

Another problem concerned the financing of health care services. Both Germany and Austria operate an insurance-based health care system that provides benefits-in-kind services to patients. In both countries sickness funds pay providers directly for medical treatment, but there is a major difference in how these costs are calculated. Austrian providers charge sickness funds only the costs of the treatment itself (based on a modified diagnosis-related group system). The charges do not include costs of operating the infrastructure or possible budget deficits; a regional Austrian health fund financed by taxation covers these. When German patients receive treatment on an Austrian hospital ward, therefore, the Austrian hospital charges the German sickness funds via an official tariff that covers both the treatment and the cost that would have been covered by taxes in Austria. As a result, the cost to German sickness funds is nearly double the cost to Austrian ones. In reaction to this, the German sickness funds announced that they would only give authorization for patients' treatment if the cost did not exceed the charge to an Austrian sickness fund. In reality, there was no reduction in bills – although no explanation was given for this – and costs remained the same until the end of the project (Interview 2).

Stakeholder roles

Various stakeholders had diverse roles at different times during the collaboration between KH Braunau and KKH Simbach. Initially, for example, the Bavarian sickness funds were major proponents of emergency care cooperation, but their leading role lessened as the project developed and the individual hospital managers filled the gap. Regional political support (and the potential lack thereof) also began to play a part. Further incentives for cross-border cooperation were the need for reorganization, significant competition and pricing pressures, and the effort to optimize regional medical services (Interview 1). Given the evolution of the project, it seems that reforms and reorganization pressures played an ambivalent role: they offered incentives for cooperation but created insurmountable obstacles, leading eventually to the termination of the project.

The context of regional governance and reforms surrounding KH Braunau initially served as an incentive for cooperation. While framework legislation on the inpatient sector is regulated at the national level in Austria, the regions (Bundesländer) are responsible for the implementation and precise regulation of hospital care. Reforms introduced at the time of the project aimed to curb the steady rise of public expenditure on health care. Rationalization measures were put in place to improve the structure of financing and the nationwide planning of hospital infrastructure (Hofmarcher and Rack, 2006). According to the Austrian Court of Auditors, smaller hospitals run the highest risk of lacking cost–effectiveness (Rechnungshof, 2010); as a consequence, the smaller Austrian hospitals located near the borders of the country came under particular pressure to increase their efficiency in inpatient care provision. This context of health care reform therefore created incentives for providers such as KH Braunau to establish cross-border cooperation to enhance efficiency.

The original request by the Bavarian sickness funds to buy services from KH Braunau and the closure of several wards in KKH Simbach imply that similar pressures existed in Germany. A series of disincentives, however, raised opposition to this "national" incentive structure. One such example arose from the action of regional authorities considering themselves bound by a national framework of regulation and standard setting: Austrian authorities are responsible for the safety and standards of treatment of Austrian patients, but treating Austrian patients in German hospital wards infringes this national requirement. As a result, the regional authorities insisted that Austrian patients in the German hospital should only receive treatment from Austrian medical staff.

In response, the managers of KH Braunau and KKH Simbach developed a joint strategy, entering into talks and negotiations with their respective regional authorities to find de facto or practical solutions to overcome such obstacles. The managers tried to make sure they appeared together at all negotiations to underline the fact that, despite differences in territorial conceptions of health care provision, both hospitals fully supported the collaboration. This international – or, more precisely, European – negotiation strategy usually facilitated their task when approaching regional authorities on both sides of the border. Both managers also made sure they extended invitations to regional politicians on a regular basis.

> "When the press called us ... we always made sure we had a unified approach. And people noticed quite quickly that they faced something unified. ... We also got appointments quicker either in the Federal Ministry of Health in Vienna or with the regional Governor in Linz. ... When we brought the German District Administrator with us, it became a political visit and then there were photos with the politicians."
>
> (Interview 1)

This strategy was successful in extending cooperation throughout the years, as the hospital managers felt that politicians were very pro-European in both regions. Regional politicians tended to support cross-border initiatives in general, but at the same time seemed surprised that practical disincentives existed. Thus, gaining regional involvement and support was crucial at each problematic point during the collaboration.

In search of further support for their cooperation, the project partners involved other national stakeholders. When the KH Braunau manager contacted the Federal Ministry of Health in Vienna to gain the support of the head of the legal affairs section, the latter suggested a solution regarding the employment contracts of seconded doctors, and also offered advice on some of the other practical aspects of the collaboration. A draft bill aimed to change the federal

Austrian framework law on hospital operations; this provided for the possibility of opening "dislodged" wards in hospitals of neighbouring countries, provided Austrian medical standards and the financing system were respected (BMGF, 2006).

Discussions during the parliamentary process of passing the law, however, revealed the limitations of highlighting the European "added value" of the existing collaboration. The bill threatened the national interests of other stakeholders in the health care system. Representatives of the Austrian Association of Private Hospitals and Medical Association in particular made it clear that a law facilitating cross-border cooperation could have unwanted side-effects: they feared that it could lead to the recruitment of doctors from neighbouring eastern European EU Member States on lower salaries. As a consequence the scope of the law diminished, allowing cross-border cooperation in the hospital sector only in an area close to the border. For the manager of KH Braunau this meant that the law became more of an obstacle than a help. Before the law came into effect the project partners could ask regional officials for exceptional permission to treat Austrian and German patients within a common structure because there were no regulations covering this area; this legal void made a pragmatic approach possible. Afterwards, however, tight legal provisions that did not allow any exceptions bound officials (Interview 1). A strategy aimed at facilitating cross-border cooperation instead limited such activities, as other national stakeholders' interests effectively circumscribed the regional actors' room for manoeuvre.

An Austrian official responsible for the inpatient sector at the regional health fund confirmed that cross-border cooperation definitely "made sense", but highlighted the territorial conception of hospital planning the fund had to follow.

"Austrian hospitals are planned for Austrian patients: if there is an influx of foreign patients this has to be integrated. But in general such cooperation is positive, where they say this is one region that connects geographically and where no true border exists anymore."

(Interview 3)

From 2010 the project partners planned to reinforce the cross-border collaboration by extending it to several other hospitals. This intensification seemed, however, to go too far in the eyes of regional authorities. The reform context, which had been favourable for cooperation, became an obstacle as the authorities decided to make hospital capacities within the region of Upper Austria more efficient. In June 2011, the regional government developed a new hospital strategy as projections predicted that hospital costs would increase significantly. In 2010 hospital funding spending was €1.7 billion; this was expected to rise to

€2.7 billion by 2020. The reform aimed to save €336 million per year. The plans included a cutback of around 700 beds in all regional hospitals, and several Upper Austrian hospitals would have either to close or to merge wards; some of these would also become day clinics (Meinhart, 2011). KH Braunau had to transform its urology and ophthalmology wards into day clinics and reduce the 419 beds in the remaining wards by 33 (Land Oberösterreich, 2011b). By the end of 2011, KH Braunau also had to close the jointly founded COR GmbH, despite its previous investment in the organization.

Pressure for reform from the regional authorities left no latitude for individual hospitals' attempts at cross-border cooperation and the Braunau–Simbach collaboration was terminated. While in 2006 Upper Austrian authorities had proudly announced the collaboration's incorporation into regional hospital planning (Landeskorrespondenz, 2006), in 2011 they claimed that the joint coronary angiography unit would conflict with "precise planning of regional hospital provision" (Landeskorrespondenz, 2011), and a spokesperson stated that "an Upper Austrian hospital should mainly serve patients from its own country" (MeinBezirk.at, 2011). Local politicians and stakeholders involved in the hospitals tried to challenge the reforms, even collecting signatures from Bavarian citizens for a petition in support of KH Braunau, but these efforts failed (UNS, 2011). A petition against the reform from the citizens of Braunau also collected 53 000 signatures, but did not change the authorities' decision (OÖNachrichten, 2011).

Role of the EU

The Austrian and German health care providers tried to eliminate or solve the problems they encountered using two strategies. The first was at the (bi-) national level described above, but given the inherent limitations of trying to gain national support, the collaboration partners also turned to the European level to intensify their cooperation, trying to make use of resources provided by the EU. These strategies were closely linked, and both partners played the "Europe card" to legitimize their efforts in talks with their respective national administrations. The Austrian discussions about regulating a European cross-border project show that cooperation is not only dependent on regional political support but also closely linked to other interests at the national level. The freedoms provided by the EU's common market, however, are not always perceived as an advantage; they can also be interpreted as a threat.

To access the investment necessary to guarantee barrier-free access for patients at both hospitals, the partners applied to the European Structural Fund. The project received roughly €200 000, which was used to set up a scheme for regular patient transport between KKH Simbach and KH Braunau and for medical coordination between the sites (Interview 3). This amount of funding played a limited role, especially compared with KH Braunau's investment in the coronary angiography unit. Nevertheless, given the duration and scope of the collaboration, the involvement of the Fund conferred a European legitimacy on the project, as the name given to the proposed "European clinical centre" indicates.

The hospital managers also tried to contact their local representatives in the European Parliament to outline their concerns about the different legal requirements in the two countries. For example, in 2007 the Bavarian Member of the European Parliament addressed a written question to the European Commission, pointing out the obstacles to cooperation arising from Austrian personnel requirements and asking for support (Weber, 2007). Despite this effort the managers felt that they were not sufficiently important players in the political process and that lobbying structures at the European level were beyond their reach.

The EU thus played two roles in the Braunau–Simbach collaboration. The first was a financial one: European funding – albeit at a limited level in this case – helped with the implementation of measures necessary to make the project work. The second role, however, seemed the more important: association with the EU expanded and legitimized the collaboration. References to its European nature facilitated and enhanced access to regional and national policy-makers and gave the project greater legitimacy in the eyes of the regional public. Nevertheless, because of its position at the regional level of governance, the collaboration had only limited direct access to the higher levels of politics in Brussels. Furthermore, the national interests of other stakeholders limited the project's potential scope once it tried to expand beyond its regional scale. In particular, as the project's development shows, national and regional pressures on health care reform, although initially presenting an incentive for cross-border cooperation, also set the general context of the collaboration in both countries. As a result, despite several years of successful cooperation and EU backing, the project was terminated.

Conclusion

The cross-border collaboration between the German KKH Simbach and the Austrian KH Braunau, initiated externally at the request of Bavarian sickness funds in 1994, soon gained pace. There were four phases of cooperation (Table 3.3). In the first, a phase of "general cooperation", the hospitals exchanged single services. After five years a second phase formalized the existing collaboration and increased its scope. One hospital rented wards from another through a lease contract, and patients of two nationalities could access medical treatment in the same structure from 2004. The third phase, "Europeanization", began after ten years of cooperation. From 2010 the project partners had planned to reinforce the cross-border collaboration by extending it to several other hospitals. This intensification and expansion of the project seems, however, to have gone too far in the eyes of the regional authorities. Eventually, German hospital restructuring and health care reforms in Upper Austria led to the project's termination.

Table 3.3. *Phases of the collaboration project*

Phase	Activity	Initiative taken by
1. General cooperation and exchange of services (from 1994)	Emergency care for trauma surgical patients and paediatric treatment: agreement between Bavarian sickness funds and KH Braunau	Germany
	Collaboration of regional emergency rescue dispatch centres	Austria and Germany
	CT scans at KH Braunau for KKH Simbach patients	Austria
2. Lease contract (from 1999)	2004–2005: relocation of two internal medicine wards from KH Braunau to KKH Simbach	Austria
3. Internationalization and "Europeanization" (from 2005)	2005: European dimension added with the EU-funded "Braunau–Simbach European clinical centre" project	Austria and Germany
	2008: creation of a joint coronary angiography unit, managed by both hospitals	Austria and Germany
	Plans to extend cross-border cooperation to more hospitals in the border region: development of a regional concept for cross-border exchange of services	Austria and Germany
Termination (2011)	Political developments on both sides of the border terminate cooperation (with the exception of emergency treatment)	Austria and Germany

While European funding did not play a dominant part in the project, the EU's role expanded and legitimized the collaboration and facilitated contact within the political arena. This was necessary to overcome several obstacles that arose from national or territorial conceptions of health care delivery, as illustrated by the examples above concerning building regulations and the national political discussion of legal initiatives to facilitate cross-border hospital cooperation. Projects positioned at the local level of governance, however, have only limited access to the political arena in Brussels to pursue lobbying activities. The same holds true with access to the national level of politics. These limits on strategic action became evident once the project entered its third phase and its scope began to reach beyond the regional level: the interests of other national stakeholders reduced its room for manoeuvre.

Analysis of the development of this collaboration between Austrian and German hospitals shows how providers at national peripheries can aim to address the needs of the local population and optimize regional health care provision. More generally, however, this case study illustrates that national and regional pressures on health care reform aiming at increased efficiency play an ambivalent role: they can present incentives for cross-border cooperation, but have the opposite effect on regional level and national stakeholders. Exploration of stakeholder interests and the role of the EU in the collaboration between KH Braunau and KKH Simbach reveals a clash between layers of interest at different levels of governance. While EU support expanded room for manoeuvre through various resources, the incentives and disincentives for such cross-border cooperation were mainly determined by national and regional reform efforts and by other national stakeholders' interests. Even though local stakeholders tried to resist, the project was eventually terminated, despite more than 18 years of successful collaboration. The example of cross-border cooperation between KH Braunau and KKH Simbach shows how the lowest (local) and highest (EU) levels of decision-making share common interests, but are not strong enough to oppose the "real" decision-makers at the regional and national levels.

References

BMGF (2006). *Entwurf – Bundesgesetz, mit dem das Bundesgesetz über Krankenanstalten und Kuranstalten und das Ärztegesetz 1998 geändert warden.* Vienna, Bundesministerium für Gesundheit und Frauen (www.parlament.gv.at/PAKT/VHG/XXII/ME/ME_00378/imfname_055607.pdf, accessed 10 June 2013).

Braunauer Spitalsmagazin [internal hospital magazine of KH Braunau], March 2011.

Braunauer Spitalsmagazin [internal hospital magazine of KH Braunau], June 2011.

Burger R, Wieland M, eds. (2010a). *healthacross Report I.* Vienna, Gesundheitsmanagement OG (www.healthacross.eu/fileadmin/ root_healthacross/healthacross/results/HA_REPORT_I.pdf, accessed 10 June 2013).

Burger R, Wieland M, eds. (2010b). *healthacross Report II.* Vienna, Gesundheitsmanagement OG (www.healthacross.eu/fileadmin/ root_healthacross/healthacross/results/healthacross_REPORT_II_.pdf, accessed 10 June 2013).

Franziskanerinnen von Vöcklabruck (2011). *Geschäftsbericht 2010.* Vöcklabruck, Franziskanerinnen von Vöcklabruck (www.franziskanerinnen.at/ gesundheit/geschaeftsbericht2010.pdf, accessed 10 June 2013).

Hofmarcher MM, Rack HM (2006). Austria: health system review. *Health Systems in Transition,* 8(3): 1–247 (www.euro.who.int/__data/assets/ pdf_file/0009/96435/E89021.pdf, accessed 10 June 2013).

Land Oberösterreich (2011a). Spitalsreform II: *"Reform nach Maß – der Oö. Weg bis 2020".* Linz, Land Oberösterreich (www.land-oberoesterreich.gv.at/ cps/rde/xbcr/SID-54C57771-768E77B9/ooe/Spitalsreform(1).pdf, accessed 10 June 2013).

Land Oberösterreich (2011b). Krankenhaus Braunau [web site]. Linz, Land Oberösterreich (www.land-oberoesterreich.gv.at/cps/rde/xchg/ SID-AF34FD4A-4EE9F997/ooe/hs.xsl/kh_braunau_DEU_HTML.htm, accessed 10 June 2013).

Landeskorrespondenz (2006). LR Stöger beauftragte Regionalen Strukturplan Gesundheit Oberösterreich 2010. *Landeskorrespondenz* 176, 1 August 2006 (www.land-oberoesterreich.gv.at/cps/rde/xchg/ooe/ hs.xsl/49938_DEU_HTML.htm, accessed 11 June 2013).

Landeskorrespondenz (2011). Spitalsreform: Panikmache durch das KH Braunau nicht angebracht – Vorschläge der Expertenkommission garantieren eine ausgezeichnete medizinische Versorgung im Innviertel. *Landeskorrespondenz* 69, 8 April 2011 (www.land-oberoesterreich.gv.at/cps/ rde/xchg/ooe/hs.xsl/103900_DEU_HTML.htm, accessed 11 June 2013).

MeinBezirk.at (2011). Behandlung deutscher Patienten eingestellt. *MeinBezirk.at* [online], 1 December (www.meinbezirk.at/braunau-am-inn/ wirtschaft/behandlung-deutscher-patienten-eingestellt-d118407.html, accessed 10 June 2013).

Meinhart G (2011). Oberösterreich: Widerstand gegen Spitalsreform. *Die Presse,* 5 April (http://diepresse.com/home/panorama/oesterreich/647897/ Oberoesterreich_Widerstand-gegen-Spitalsreform, accessed 10 June 2013).

OÖNachrichten (2011). Spitalsreform: 90.000 Proteste, Sondersitzung. *nachrichten.at* [online], 4 May (www.nachrichten.at/oberoesterreich/ innviertel/art70,613150, accessed 11 June 2013).

Rechnungshof (2010). *Verwaltungsreform: Problemanalyse Gesundheit und Pflege.* Vienna, Der Rechnungshof (www.rechnungshof.gv.at/ fileadmin/downloads/2010/beratung/verwaltungsreform/Gesundheit/ Problemanalyse_Gesundheit_und_Pflege.pdf, accessed 10 June 2013).

Rottal-Inn Kliniken (2012). Pressemitteilung: 03.02.2012: Herzkatheter jetzt auch für Notfälle [web site]. Eggenfelden, Rottal-Inn Kliniken (www.rottalinnkliniken.de/aktuell/presse/archiv/2012/presse-archiv-2012. php?oid=121, accessed 10 June 2013).

UNS (2011). Spitalsreform bedeutet auch weitere Verschlechterung der medizinischen Versorgung der Bevölkerung von Simbach und dem Inntal [web site]. Simbach, Unabhängige Simbacher Bürgerliste – UNS (http://uns-in-simbach.de/110502.htm, accessed 11 June 2013).

Weber, M (2007). *"Europaklinik" in Simbach–Braunau: written question by Manfred Weber (PPE-DE) to the Commission*, P-2657/07, 15 May (www.europarl.europa.eu/sides/getDoc.do?pubRef=-%2f%2fEP%2f%2f TEXT%2bWQ%2bP-2007-2657%2b0%2bDOC%2bXML%2bV0%2f%2fE N&language=EN, accessed 11 June 2013).

Annex 3.1 Interviews conducted

Number	Date	Interviewee	Institution
Interview 1	9 September 2009	Erwin Windischbauer, Financial and Administrative Director	Hospital St Josef Braunau, Braunau
Interview 2	12 January 2011	Erwin Windischbauer, Financial and Administrative Director	Hospital St Josef Braunau, Braunau
Interview 3	29 October 2010	Stefan Potyka, Head of Unit, Unit for Inpatient Care	Upper Austrian Health Fund, Linz

Strategic positioning and creative solutions: French patient flows to hospitals and polyclinics in the Belgian Ardennes (Belgium–France)

Régine Kiasuwa and Rita Baeten

Introduction

The Ardennes region covers a rural area in the south-east of Belgium and north-east of France. On the French side, the territory around the Meuse River with the town of Givet at its centre – commonly called "la botte de Givet" [the boot of Givet] – is surrounded by Belgium. The activity of two local hospitals in this French enclave was, for economic reasons, drastically reduced from 2002 onwards; as a result, the nearest hospital offering a full range of health care services was 60 km away. Under pressure from the local population, policy-makers and field actors looked for innovative solutions to compensate for the lack of care provision on the French side. Successive agreements were developed to allow French citizens with social health insurance (SHI) in la botte de Givet to be treated across the border in the nearby Belgian hospital at Dinant (CH de Dinant). This resulted in significant and mostly one-way patient flows from France to Belgium.

This chapter examines these developments and investigates why the initial hospital collaboration, instigated and controlled by the health authorities, turned into one between competing health insurers and hospitals across the border. It describes the context, origins and operation of the collaboration and the scale of patient flows; analyses the stakes of all actors involved to understand why the collaboration occurred and what incentives it created; and explores the role of the European Union (EU) in the project. Accepting the rationale of ensuring access to local health care services for the population of the Ardennes region, the analysis shows how the area became a laboratory of experimental cross-border collaboration and how the incentives for stakeholders created a dynamic in which they applied legal frameworks in a very creative way. Practical arrangements, negotiations and tacit agreements decided between field actors eventually became the project's modus operandi, often before any legal basis existed or in spite of existing ones.

Methodology

The authors carried out desk research to understand the context of the collaboration, develop an overview of the differences between the Belgian and French health care systems, identify the main actors and collect data (about flows and legal frameworks). They also conducted 12 semi-structured face-to-face interviews with 18 field actors in both countries, working with a grid drafted specifically for each interview (see Annex 4.1 for interview details).

Interviewee selection took place with the aim of covering a wide range of positions, including hospital administrators, sickness fund representatives, members of regional and national public authorities and health care professionals from both sides of the border. The authors also requested interviews with the six French health care facilities involved, three French general practitioners (GPs) and one gynaecologist in the Ardennes but received no response. The authors recorded and fully transcribed seven of the interviews, drafting summaries for the remaining five. Interviewees also provided additional relevant documents and data.

To process the material, the authors coded the interviews. They also developed a written questionnaire; this was distributed by the secretariat of the gynaecology unit to 88 French women who had given birth in CH de Dinant, during their postnatal visit. The women sent back 14 completed (anonymous) questionnaires.

Context and evolution of the Ardennes collaboration

The region and its health care facilities

The Ardennes region has similar characteristics on both sides of the border. It is a mainly rural area with low and decreasing population density and an ageing population. The French territory of la botte de Givet around the river Meuse is a land strip of 21 000 inhabitants (INSEE, 2012) surrounded by Belgium (Map 4.1). On the French side the population's socioeconomic status and health status are relatively low (Interview 5).

Map 4.1. *The French–Belgian border (la botte de Givet circled)*

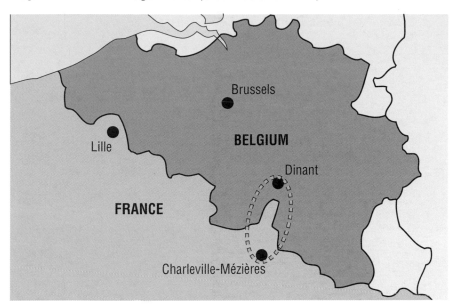

Source: Observatoire social européen.

La botte de Givet is in the French department of Ardennes, part of Champagne-Ardenne – one of France's 27 regions – where the density of health care providers and facilities is below the national average (Table 4.1). Because of the region's low population density and impoverished socioeconomic situation, local hospitals often find it difficult to attract specialists (Interviews 5 and 6).

Table 4.1. *Density of health care providers in Champagne-Ardenne and France, 2009*

Resources	Number per 10 000 inhabitants	
	Champagne-Ardenne	France
GPs	102.1	109.5
Self-employed nurses	75.8	120.2
Places (hospitalization beds and day care)	10.9	16.6

Source: INSEE, 2010.

Another French hospital, which has about 650 beds and a wide range of specialties, is CH de Charleville-Mézières (Map 4.2). The towns of Givet and Charleville-Mézières are about 60 km apart, via a two-lane secondary road cut deep into a mountainous landscape: the journey takes at least one hour. On the other side of the border, CH de Dinant, located 15 km from Givet, offers an almost complete range of health care services.

Map 4.2. *Distribution of hospitals in the Ardennes border region*

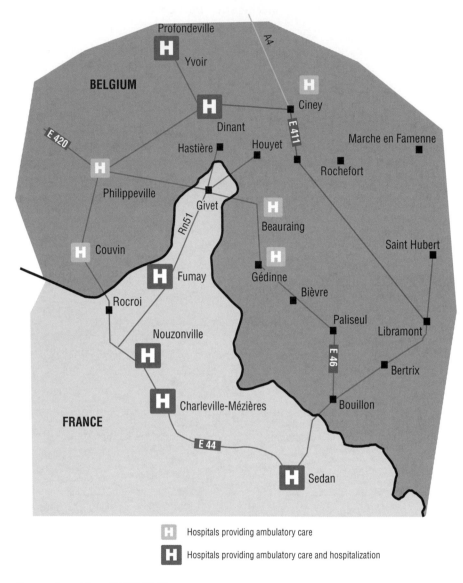

Hospitals providing ambulatory care

Hospitals providing ambulatory care and hospitalization

Source: adapted from OFBS, 2013.

Origins of the collaboration

Health care collaboration along the French–Belgian border began in the 1990s. Hospitals set up agreements giving socially insured people in a defined border area access to specific hospitals across the border for particular treatments.

Since 1995 French and Belgian health care facilities and sickness funds have signed seven inter-hospital agreements. The Observatoire Franco-Belge de la santé [Franco-Belgian Health Observatory] (OFBS), co-funded by consecutive EU Interreg programmes,[1] initiated most of these cooperation projects (Interview 7). The OFBS was created in 1999, at the initiative of sickness funds from both sides of the border, with the aim of organizing cross-border access to care. It now has more than 60 members, including health care providers, public authorities and health insurers.

As a general rule, EU regulations on the coordination of social security systems govern the funding of care for patients who go abroad for treatment.[2] Within this framework, patients need an E112 form from the health service or sickness fund in their country of origin as authorization to visit another EU Member State for treatment. In 2000, the "Transcards" project was set up in the Thiérache border region adjacent to the Ardennes; this was the first system to allow automatic delivery of the E112 form (Interview 2). The project, which was financially supported by the EU (initially by the European Commission's Directorate-General for Employment and Social Affairs and later by Interreg iii), was a success and supported local demand to establish a simpler administrative system for cross-border patients.

When the maternity service at the French clinic in Revin closed in 2002, the mayor of Givet engaged to find a solution that would spare pregnant women the 60 km drive to CH de Charleville-Mézières to give birth. In 2002–2003, these women received an E112 form from their SHI fund, CPAM des Ardennes, which allowed them to give birth in the Belgian CH de Dinant. The arrangement initially applied only to deliveries, but at the request of the women, and to ensure continuity of care, subsequently also included pre- and postnatal follow-up care (Interview 3).

When the clinic at Givet also closed in 2004, the need to create a more structured solution arose. The mayor of Givet and the Champagne-Ardenne Regional Hospital Agency (replaced by the Regional Health Agency in 2010)

---

1   The Interreg programmes aim to stimulate cross-border cooperation between regions in the EU. They started in 1989 and are financed by the European Regional Development Fund (ERDF).

2   Regulation (EC) No 883/2004 of the European Parliament and of the Council of 29 April 2004 on the coordination of social security systems. *Official Journal of the European Union*, L 166: 1–123 (http://eur-lex.europa.eu/LexUriServ/ LexUriServ.do?uri=OJ:L:2004:166:0001:0123:en:PDF, accessed 17 June 2013) and Regulation (EC) No 987/2009 of the European Parliament and of the Council of 16 September 2009 laying down the procedure for implementing Regulation (EC) No 883/2004 on the coordination of social security systems. *Official Journal of the European Union*, L 284: 1–42 (http://eur-lex.europa.eu/LexUriServ/LexUriServ.do?uri=OJ:L:2009:284:0001:0042:EN:PDF, accessed 17 June 2013).

came up with an innovative proposal: to regard CH de Dinant as a branch of CH de Charleville-Mézières for the purposes of health care payments. On 15 June 2004, the Champagne-Ardenne Regional Hospital Agency, CH de Charleville-Mézières and CH de Dinant signed a joint agreement; this also involved CPAM des Ardennes, although not as a signatory party for legal reasons. The scheme allowed French patients from Givet and Fumay to be hospitalized in CH de Dinant for internal medicine, obstetrics and surgery, and to be treated as if they were in France (Interview 3). CH de Dinant thus became a de facto part of the health care system in Champagne-Ardenne.

Unlike most other collaboration initiatives on the French–Belgian border, EU regulations on the coordination of social security systems did not govern payments under this scheme. Instead, CH de Dinant sent the bills for French patients to CH de Charleville-Mézières, which recoded the invoices and transmitted them to CPAM des Ardennes as if the patient had received treatment in France. The French hospital then transferred the SHI fund payments to the Belgian hospital. Some members of the region's population put pressure on their sickness funds and local politicians to expand the arrangement to cover ambulatory care, but without success: the agreement did not comply with existing legal frameworks in Belgium and in France so there was no legal basis for the amendment.

A bilateral framework agreement between France and Belgium,[3] signed in 2005 and in force from 2011 once ratified by France in 2007 and by Belgium in 2010, provided the legal basis for further cooperation (Box 4.1). This resulted from the French government's concern that local actors were setting up initiatives on cross-border care and signing agreements without providing information to central ministries, while a series of issues concerning such agreements could only be resolved through the involvement of national authorities. The agreement therefore provided a fixed structure for creating specific local agreements with hospitals and health authorities, with a uniform method of implementation (Harant, 2006).

Following the creation of this framework agreement, the Champagne-Ardenne regional health care plan of 2006 stipulated that CH de Dinant was integrated into the region's health care system, in order to offer local hospital care to the populations of Givet and Fumay (ARH de Champagne-Ardenne, 2006).

---

3 Accord cadre entre le Gouvernement du Royaume de Belgique et le Gouvernement de la République française sur la cooperation sanitaire transfrontalière, signée à Mouscron le 30 septembre 2005. *Moniteur Belge*, 18.02.2011: 11910 (http://reflex.raadvst-consetat.be/reflex/pdf/Mbbs/2011/02/18/118279.pdf, accessed 14 June 2013).

Box 4.1. *Framework agreement between France and Belgium on cross-border health cooperation*

The objectives of the agreement are (1) to ensure better access to high-quality health care for people living in the border area; (2) to ensure continuity of care for these populations; (3) to optimize the organization of health care provision by facilitating the use or sharing of human and material resources; (4) to promote the exchange of knowledge and best practices.

The agreement defines the bodies and organizations authorized to sign contracts for cross-border cooperation between health care facilities in border areas and the zones at both sides of the border where the agreement applies. These contracts can arrange cooperation between existing health care facilities and resources, and can create organizations for cooperation or set up joint facilities.

Based on the agreement, an "administrative arrangement" defines those authorized to sign contracts. On the French side this includes the Direction Régionale des Affaires Sanitaires et Sociales, the Regional Hospital Agency (replaced by the Regional Health Agency in 2010) and regional associations for SHI; on the Belgian side it includes the National Institute for Health and Disability Insurance (NIHDI), sickness funds and health care providers. This administrative arrangement also stipulates that if the Belgian authorities are not involved in the negotiation they must be notified prior to the signing of any contract.

The agreement stipulates that any contract must include terms and conditions for intervention for health care facilities, social security organizations and health professionals; financial details; and guarantees of continuity of patient care. It also confirms that EU regulations on the coordination of social security systems apply for payment of care received abroad, and that if prior authorization is required, the appropriate institution will issue it automatically. Nevertheless, contracts can stipulate direct payment by the health insurance company, according to specific agreed tariffs approved by the appropriate national authorities, or payment based on the tariffs of the country of affiliation, on application of Court of Justice of the European Union case law.

The agreement also stipulates that existing contracts must be adapted to comply with the framework agreement.

On the basis of the agreement, the OFBS set up six "zones organisées d'accès aux soins transfrontaliers" [organized cross-border areas for access to care] (ZOASTs) at the French–Belgian border, under the EU Interreg iv programme. A specific agreement delineating the geographical areas concerned and the conditions for benefiting from the system regulates each of these areas (ASMUP 08, 2008; Box 4.2). The ZOAST system draws on the existing cooperation projects for cross-border health care mentioned above.

Box 4.2. *ZOAST Ardennes agreement*

This agreement came into force in 2008 and has undergone several amendments. After the framework agreement between France and Belgium (Box 4.1) came into force in 2011, the ZOAST Ardennes agreement was aligned with it in early 2012. The following parties are signatories to the current version of the agreement (January 2012):

- in France, the Champagne-Ardenne Regional Health Agency;

- in Belgium, CH de Dinant, the university hospital at Mont Godinne, the polyclinics of the socialist sickness fund (for ambulatory care) and CH Santé des Fagnes of Chimay, as well as the seven Belgian sickness funds.

The agreement applies to the following health care facilities:

- in Belgium, the hospital signatories and their polyclinics;

- in France, CH de Charleville-Mézières, CH de Sedan, the local hospital at Fumay, the polyclinic of Parc de Charleville, the clinic of Dr l'Hoste at Villers-Serneuse, the polyclinic at Nouzonville and the university hospital at Reims (the regional referral centre).

The agreement, which applies for an unlimited duration, authorizes reimbursement for care provided in one of the designated health care facilities across the border for all socially insured people residing in the ZOAST in both countries (regardless of their SHI scheme). All types of care are included, both inpatient and outpatient, except medically assisted reproduction.

EU regulations on the coordination of social security systems are the basis for care payments. To this end, patients receive a specific authorization form – a so-called "administrative E112" form – a posteriori.

The contracting parties commit to provide a detailed assessment report annually to the appropriate authorities, including statistical and financial information.

The health insurance company to which the patient is affiliated covers out-of-pocket payments for French patients who benefit from 100% statutory cover. This cover does not include private room supplements.

Source: ASMUP 08, 2008.

The ZOAST Ardennes agreement in practice

The agreement, in force from February 2008, simplified the processes of verification of patients' insurance status and issuing of the administrative E112 form, allowing patients to follow administrative access procedures similar to those in their own countries. When French patients arrive at a Belgian hospital covered by the agreement they show their national health insurance cards and reader devices in the hospital allow administrative staff to access all the required information. Through an electronic portal, and within 48 hours, the hospital receives the automatic administrative E112 form from the SHI fund to which the patient is affiliated (Interview 7).

French patients treated in Belgium for the first time require administrative affiliation to a local sickness fund. Since most French patients have no idea which of the seven qualifying sickness funds to choose, in practice the choice is made by the Belgian hospital. The two largest Belgian sickness funds, Mutualité socialiste and Mutualité chrétienne, set up an agreement with local hospitals that they would share the affiliation of French patients, alternating each month (Interviews 3 and 6).

The ZOAST Ardennes agreement made important changes to the original 2004 joint agreement. All types of inpatient and outpatient care are now included except medically assisted reproduction, which is only reimbursed in France and allowed under specific conditions that do not apply in Belgium (Interview 8); eight health care facilities and seven sickness funds are now involved on the Belgian side; and the area from which patients can cross the border is much larger (Map 4.3).

Map 4.3. *Area covered by the ZOAST Ardennes agreement*

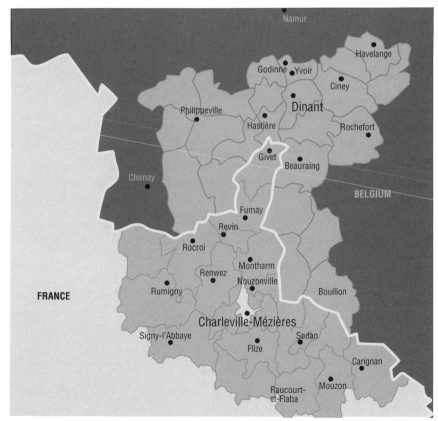

Source: adapted from OFBS, 2013.

The agreement meant the end of the hospital collaboration between CH de Charleville-Mézières and CH de Dinant since there was no longer an administrative or financial reason to collaborate: instead, the two hospitals have become competitors. Cross-border collaboration now takes place either between French and Belgian sickness funds or between sickness funds and hospitals.

Problems and solutions

Several differences between the French and Belgian health care systems generated problems for French patients going to Belgium for treatment, necessitating the development of creative solutions to address them.

In France, SHI covers about 75% of a patient's health care expenditure, although some patients have 100% coverage. What SHI does not cover can be covered fully or partly by voluntary health insurance (VHI), but reimbursement levels may vary between VHI funds. For hospital care, the provider receives direct payment for the difference. In Belgium, on the other hand, the social security system pays the larger part of hospitalization costs. Co-payments, made by the patient directly, consist of specific flat rates per day and per stay. French patients deemed the difference between these schemes an obstacle to visiting Belgium for treatment; to avoid the need for direct co-payments Belgian hospitals sent additional invoices – only for French patients – directly to their VHI funds. As of 2009, the hospitals send these invoices to one French insurer (MGEN des Ardennes) which centralizes the bills and dispatches them to other French SHI and VHI funds.

If a French patient requests a private hospital room or receives treatment from a physician who does not adhere to the collectively agreed tariffs in Belgium, the Belgian doctor can set a customized tariff for treatment. French SHI funds and most French VHI funds do not reimburse these supplements, so Belgian hospitals warn French patients to check with their VHI fund before choosing a private room (Interview 6).

French patients were also not familiar with the requirement for upfront payment for ambulatory care applicable in Belgian hospitals. To avoid payment problems and patient dissatisfaction, French insurers, Belgian insurers and Belgian hospitals tacitly agreed to apply a third-party payment system for ambulatory care – for French patients only – although this is formally forbidden by Belgian legislation (Interviews 3, 5, 6, 7 and 8).

A further obstacle was that for technical reasons French VHI funds were not able to pay foreign hospitals (Interviews 8 and 9). French patients had to pay in advance and claim reimbursement from the fund on their return to France.

To avoid this, in a pilot project two Belgian hospitals received a specific "FINESS" number, which gave them the status of official French hospitals (Interview 6). With this number, the Belgian hospitals opened bank accounts in France, into which French VHI funds pay invoices directly (Interviews 2 and 8).

Scale of cooperation

From 2002 cross-border flows for maternity care increased steadily, but in recent years the number of deliveries has stabilized (Table 4.2). In October 2011, CH de Dinant celebrated the thousandth delivery of a French baby (Interview 11).

Table 4.2. *French women delivering at CH de Dinant, 2002–2011*

Year	2002	2003	2004	2005	2006	2007[a]	2008	2009	2010	2011
Deliveries	10	54	83	121	126	114	92	131	149	137

Source: administration office of CH de Dinant.
Note: [a] In 2007 the hospital lost one gynaecologist.

Table 4.3 shows the numbers of French patients treated at CH de Dinant, distinguishing between French patients treated under the ZOAST Ardennes agreement (living in the area covered by the agreement) and French patients outside that area. The table shows a steady increase in numbers of ZOAST patients and activities since the agreement was set up. For non-ZOAST patients treated in this period the trend is less clear and the hospital provided no clarification to help understand these fluctuations.

Patients from France represent about 15% to 20% of CH de Dinant's turnover (for both ambulatory care and inpatient care): a very high proportion (Interview 3). In particular, the departments of neurology and ophthalmology receive many French patients, apparently because the waiting times are shorter than for the equivalent departments in France (Interview 3). According to data provided by the hospital the four main services sought by French patients are ophthalmology, gynaecology, radiology and paediatrics.

Table 4.3. *French patients treated and numbers of treatments at CH de Dinant, 2009–2011*

Year	Patients treated		Outpatient care units		Hospitalizations, including day hospitalization	
	ZOAST	Other	ZOAST	Other	ZOAST	Other
2009	3 468	N/A	8 837	1 778	2 634	94
2010	5 112	N/A	12 833	3 374	3 700	153
2011	6 055	N/A	15 316	294	4 073	106

Source: based on data provided by CH de Dinant.

In 2010, the university hospital of Mont Godinne treated 477 French patients for both ambulatory and inpatient care (out of a total of about 32 000 patients). Although this represents only about 1.5% of the patient population, it is an important increase compared with the 257 patients treated in 2009 (of which 64% received ambulatory care) (Interview 6). The polyclinics of the socialist sickness fund (which only provide ambulatory care) receive about 5000 French patients per year and numbers are increasing (Interview 7).

Flows of Belgian patients to France, on the other hand, are negligible. In 2009 only two Belgian patients received treatment in CH de Sedan and two in CH de Charleville-Mézières.

Stakeholder perspectives

As argued in earlier research, for cross-border collaboration to work, all actors involved need to have a stake in the project (Glinos and Baeten, 2006). The following sections examine the incentives for each group of stakeholders.

Patients

Patient flows from France to Belgium are strong first and foremost because French patients have incentives to visit Belgian hospitals. Without an objective need from patients other actors cannot encourage mobility, however much they might like to. The specific geographical situation of the ZOAST Ardennes agreement explains much about the flows: proximity seems to be the decisive factor, and 95% of French patients treated in CH de Dinant come from Givet or Fumay (Interview 8), the two towns closest to Dinant. Patients particularly appreciate the option of receiving treatment close to home while enjoying the same administrative and financial facilities as in their home country (Interviews 3, 7 and 11). They also welcome the prospect of undergoing medical examinations and receiving the results on the same day, whereas this requires several visits in France (Interview 6). Proximity, speed, efficiency and quality of services in Belgium are the main reasons put forward to explain the flows (Interviews 6, 8 and 11).

These incentives were confirmed by the French women who gave birth in CH de Dinant and filled out the patient questionnaire. The 14 respondents lived on average 30.7 km from CH de Dinant and 62.3 km from CH de Charleville-Mézières. Nine of the respondents perceived the care in CH de Dinant as being of better quality than in the French maternity unit. Belgian gynaecologists reported that most French women who had given birth in Belgium came back for all types of gynaecological care, including annual visits and follow-up

(Interview 10), even though two French gynaecologists offer consultations in la botte de Givet.

French GPs

French GPs play an important role in referring patients to Belgium. According to the interviewees, they prefer to refer their patients to CH de Dinant than to CH de Charleville-Mézières because they are pleased with the care provided in Belgium and the flow of information (Interviews 3, 6 and 11). GPs have a separate phone number that connects directly to the hospital services they want to reach without having to pass through the telephone exchange (Interviews 4 and 8). They also have direct electronic access to their patients' files at CH de Dinant and can consult examination results as soon as they are available (Interviews 3, 8 and 10).

Belgian sickness funds

The Belgian sickness funds are the main instigators of the collaboration (Interview 12). Since the 1990s the OFBS – which the sickness funds on both sides of the border originally set up – has taken the initiative in devising agreements at the French–Belgian border. The sickness funds' aim is to accumulate knowledge and experience regarding administrative procedures and to develop networks. They expect an EU health care market to open up and hope to have a competitive advantage when this happens: "Si on n'est pas sur le terrain, les autres y seront de toute façon [If we are not in the field others will be, in any case]" (Interview 7). They also receive a 7.2% supplement to cover administration costs on the invoices to French patients (Interviews 7 and 12); this is on top of the lump sum they receive for administration costs on the invoices to their Belgian affiliates.

French SHI funds

The French SHI funds are the historic allies of the Belgian sickness funds, collaborating closely with them from the beginning to allow patients access to cross-border care. Since 2009, Belgian hospitals send all bills for French patients treated in the Ardennes to CPAM des Ardennes, where they are centralized. This organization and MGEN des Ardennes (which is involved in both SHI and VHI) are the "pivot" bodies and the main intermediaries for Belgian partners (Interview 8). They plan to centralize invoicing for cross-border patients from the entire French–Belgian border (for all six ZOASTs).

Because of the scale of patient flows in the Ardennes, they have implemented new information technology equipment and programmes to manage the bills.

If they receive authorization to become the central unit for cross-border invoices on the French side these organizations will receive important funds for doing so from Caisse nationale de l'assurance maladie des travailleurs salariés (CNAMTS), the national health insurance fund, which is under the direct supervision of the Ministry of Social Security and the Ministry of Economy and Finance (Interview 8). This development would suit most actors in the field (Interview 9): Belgian stakeholders would only need to deal with one well-informed and well-equipped intermediary; the Champagne-Ardenne Regional Health Agency would have easier access to data on cross-border flows, enabling more efficient health care planning; and other French insurers would not need to adapt their information technology systems or provide extra training for their administrative staff.

French VHI funds

The ZOAST Ardennes agreement does not apply to French VHI funds. The reaction of these funds to the collaboration differs according to how many of their clients are in the Ardennes: those with high numbers are very active in setting up systems to facilitate cross-border care and to establish cross-border networks of sickness funds (Interview 4). Those with a limited number of clients in the border region are very reluctant to engage in the system and to reimburse supplements to the tariff. Of the thousands of VHI funds involved, only one third reimburse for care provided in Belgium (Interviews 3 and 8).

Because these VHI funds raised concerns that fees would be higher for treatments in Belgium (Interview 8), CPAM des Ardennes and MGEN des Ardennes provided evidence showing that the cost to the VHI fund is never greater than it is for treatment in France. They also argued that affiliates might switch to another VHI fund if they could not receive reimbursement for such fees. The system, however, remains difficult to understand and to accept for those not involved in the collaboration or located in the border area. The funds are reluctant to invest the time needed to understand and apply this complex system for just a few patients. This is another reason why MGEN des Ardennes centralizes invoices for complementary health insurance from Belgium and dispatches them to the other VHI funds.

Belgian hospitals

Belgian CH de Dinant was very motivated to treat French patients from the beginning, and engaged in major efforts to facilitate the collaboration.

In addition to important investments in software, it organized information sessions in France to reassure referring health professionals about the way the hospital runs. Belgian hospital funding depends on occupation rates, and hospitals must meet minimum activity levels. Before 2008 CH de Dinant had a relatively low occupation rate (Interview 4), but with the French patients, its activity level has increased.

The university hospital of Mont Godinne, on the other hand, receives fewer patients from France. It aims to position itself internationally as a highly technologically equipped reference centre and as the main university hospital of the region[4] (Interview 6).

French hospitals

Regional health care facilities in France are worried about these outflows of patients, fearing the potential financial consequences of losing patients. The creation of an additional agreement on emergency transport worsened the relationship between Belgian and French hospitals, since patients are increasingly transported to CH de Dinant for emergency care (Interview 4).

French health authorities and insurers believe that CH de Charleville-Mézières perceives the ZOAST Ardennes agreement and the consequent patient flows to Belgium as a threat and one of the reasons for its enormous financial deficits (Interviews 3, 6 and 9). It is perhaps no coincidence that all six French hospitals involved in the agreement declined interviews. There is currently no contact between CH de Charleville-Mézières and CH de Dinant (Interview 3).

Strikingly, whereas the ZOAST Ardennes agreement includes most municipalities of the Charleville-Mézières district, it excludes citizens of the town of Charleville-Mézières itself from access to care in Belgium (see Map 4.3). The reason advanced is that they have access to a hospital with a wide range of specialities and thus do not need the agreement (Interviews 4, 6–8 and 9).

Belgian physicians

Physicians from CH de Dinant made it clear that the initiative to treat French patients had not come from them and they had not requested the patient flows. They also claimed not to distinguish between French and Belgian patients (Interviews 10 and 11). Nevertheless, treating French patients assists specialists at a university hospital, such as the one at Mont Godinne, in building an international reputation (Interview 6).

---

4   The nearest French university hospital is located in Reims, at a distance of 150 km.

Public authorities

Authorities on both sides of the border have concerns about the increasing patient flows. When the Champagne-Ardenne Regional Health Agency signed the ZOAST Ardennes agreement it did not expect the flow to reach such high numbers in one direction (Interview 9). Indeed, in other cross-border collaboration projects at the Belgian–French border, flows are much more even in both directions. The Champagne-Ardenne Regional Health Agency is concerned that patients are going abroad for care that they could receive perfectly well in France, and fears for the future of certain health care services in Charleville-Mézières. Under a 2009 French law aiming to reform and streamline health care provision,[5] loss of patients could mean closure of services, which could put local care for people living in the Charleville-Mézières area at risk (Interview 9).

The Belgian authorities are similarly worried that the increasing patient inflow could put access to health care for local Belgian citizens at risk (Interview 12). For example, the gynaecology service of CH de Dinant is fully occupied and unable to accept new patients (Interview 10). As a consequence, new Belgian patients have to attend the next closest hospital for these services, which is some 20–30 km away.

Whereas on the French side regional public authorities are signatories of cross-border contracts, on the Belgian side only private, not-for-profit actors can sign. Nevertheless, the contracts can only enter into force in Belgium once approved by the Insurance Committee of the NIHDI, which represents all Belgian sickness funds (Interviews 2 and 12). In addition, hospitals must provide the NIHDI with information about patient flows to ensure that the contracts do not affect access to health care for domestic patients. While this information has been requested since 2004, the first data were only provided in 2010, for the year 2009 (Interview 12). The actors involved seem reluctant to provide data (on all the ZOASTs) because, according to one stakeholder, they fear that Belgian public authorities might question the efficacy of the collaborations, in particular because the very low flows from Belgium to France suggest that Belgian patients have no real need for the agreement.[6]

---

5   Law No. 2009-879 of 21 July 2009 created new legal entities called "communautés hospitalières de territoire" [local hospital communities] by regrouping a range of small and large hospitals on the basis of complementary areas of expertise.

6   Email communication from the manager of a Belgian sickness fund, 7 June 2012.

Role of the EU

When asked, most interviewees – and health care providers in particular – did not consider the EU's role in the cooperation initiative important (Interviews 3, 7 and 11), although some acknowledged the possibility that the EU creates opportunities for working on cross-border projects (Interview 7). Those most familiar with European frameworks are those in receipt of EU funding – in particular the sickness funds within the OFBS (Interviews 2, 7, 8 and 12).

Nevertheless, the EU clearly played a key role in the setting up and operation of the collaboration (MOT, 2012), and whether any of the ZOASTs would have existed without EU frameworks and programmes is debatable for several reasons. First, EU Regulation 883/2004[7] applies to payments for care received abroad. Second, the OFBS, which has benefited from EU (co-)funding under the Interreg programmes since 1999, instigated all the initiatives for cross-border cooperation at the Belgian–French border. Third, the Court of Justice of the EU rulings on patient mobility created an environment in which actors started to reflect on their position in an international instead of a national market and to deploy strategies to anticipate the opening of borders for health care. Fourth, local actors use the EU to legitimize their initiatives and to convince and impress other stakeholders. Fig. 4.1 shows an insurer's invoice to a VHI fund, containing EU logos with the aim of encouraging the reimbursement of cross-border care, even though this bill has no direct connection with the EU.

Local actors manage most practical arrangements and make very creative use of existing frameworks. As a result, they sometimes perceive the EU legal framework as irrelevant and too far removed from reality (Interviews 3, 6 and 8). Many stressed in interview that non-field actors, who are not aware of the situation on the ground, design these legal settings. For instance, they criticized the fact that the EU Regulation only applies to SHI and not to VHI funds (Interview 8), which can cause problems for French patients.

Some stakeholders urged caution towards EU law in interviews; they feared that opening borders could harm public health.

> "Il ne faut pas faire de la santé un bien comme un autres, ce n'est pas du tout le cas. La ZOAST c'est intelligent, parce que c'est la création d'une zone de liberté encadrée [We should not make health a commodity like any other ... The ZOAST is a clever construction: its strength is that it creates a well-framed zone of freedom]."
>
> (Interview 6)

---

7   Regulation (EC) No 883/2004 on the coordination of social security systems (see Origins of the collaboration section, Note 2).

Some also felt that the EU and health care field actors were not working towards the same goal.

> "La cour de justice est pour la libéralization qui déstructurerait nos services nationaux. Ici, on veut vraiment une complémentarité de terrain et une mise en accord des systèmes qui gèrent la sécurité sociale et pas une uniformité de l'Europe [The Court of Justice of the European Union is in favour of liberalization, which would deconstruct our national services. Here, we want real complementarity and agreements between services that manage social security, not European uniformity]."
>
> (Interview 7)

Fig. 4.1. *Invoice from MGEN to a VHI fund*

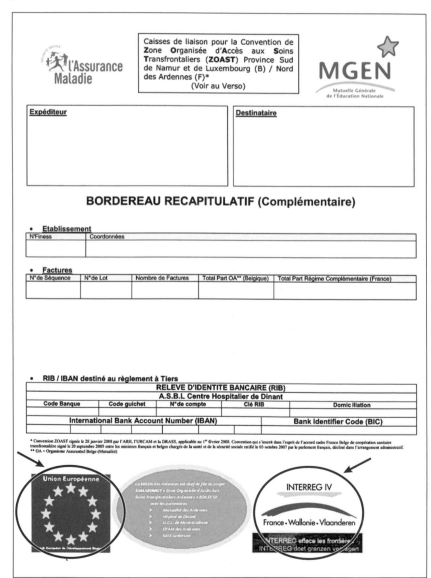

Consequences of the agreement

Competition

Sickness funds play a leading role in this collaboration. The bigger French and Belgian health insurers (both SHI and VHI) are trying to maintain their monopoly on handling cross-border patient files. By investing heavily in the project they hope to position themselves for the future.

The ZOAST Ardennes agreement's entry into force in 2008 transformed cross-border collaboration between hospitals into competition. Under the earlier hospital financing scheme, French health care facilities received a mainly prospective budget and did not have much financial responsibility, meaning that they had few incentives to increase competition, quality of service and efficiency. By contrast, the Belgian hospital landscape is highly competitive as a result of an oversupply of health care services and largely performance-based hospital funding. The management culture of the French public hospitals, less used to working in a competitive environment, encourages French patients to visit private hospitals and facilitates their choice of Belgian providers. The French public hospitals involved in the ZOAST Ardennes agreement seem to perceive the increasing competition it provokes as a threat. Nevertheless, according to French stakeholders, a new activity-based hospital funding system introduced in France in 2007, combined with domestic competition between private and public hospitals, is more to blame for the precarious financial position and deficits of French public hospitals in the region than the outflows of patients to Belgium (Interview 9).

Outside the legal frameworks

The high level of competition between hospitals and among sickness funds led stakeholders to come up with many inventive responses to practical issues, making creative use of existing (or absent) frameworks and arranging solutions that were not in accordance with the legislation in force. First, the 2004 joint agreement through which CH de Dinant became a branch of CH de Charleville-Mézières did not comply with existing legal frameworks, even though French local authorities were involved; it was created because the authorities had to meet population needs while maintaining control over patient flows. Second, insurers and Belgian hospitals had a tacit agreement to apply a third-party payment system for ambulatory care, contrary to Belgian legislation (Interviews 4 and 6). A third illustration is the inappropriate use of the former E111 form or the current European Health Insurance Card (EHIC).

These forms aim to provide citizens with access to health care services that become medically necessary during a temporary stay abroad. Although it is clear that the card is not valid for planned care abroad, several stakeholders reported that French patients living outside the area of the ZOAST Ardennes agreement are increasingly visiting Belgian hospitals to receive treatment with their EHIC (Interviews 3, 5, 7 and 9). Furthermore, patients came to Belgium with their E111 forms before 2008 for treatments not included in the ZOAST Ardennes agreement: to ensure that treatment would take place, patients needed to know that their EHIC would be accepted and health care providers needed to be sure that they would be reimbursed by sickness funds. An implicit accord between these actors was required at minimum to implement such unofficial practices.

Power struggles between field actors and health authorities

On both sides of the border, local and national authorities have to grant field actors authorization before they can make practical arrangements. Most of the time, however, agreements are set up first and are only afterwards – and not always – presented to the appropriate authority.

A planned polyclinic in Givet, where Belgian and French physicians would work together, is illustrative in this regard. The facility was proposed by CH de Dinant and is supported by Belgian and French health insurers and other Belgian hospitals. All stakeholders seem very enthusiastic about the project, which according to them is almost ready to launch (Interview 8). It was therefore a great surprise to learn from the Champagne-Ardenne Regional Health Agency that no one had submitted an application to open this polyclinic, and that even if a request had been tendered it would probably not have received authorization (Interview 9). Similar surprises also exist on the Belgian side. The NIHDI did not know that field actors had decided to implement a third-party payment system that did not comply with the law, and was also unaware that only two Belgian sickness funds dealt with the administration of cross-border patients' files (Interview 12).

National authorities on both sides of the border tried to rein in practices such as tacit agreements on the edge of the law set up between local actors. An example of an initiative from the French side is the "Contrat local de santé" [local health contract] project, put forward in 2010 to local hospitals in the Transcards region by the two French regional health agencies of du Nord and Nord-Pas-de-Calais. The goal was to optimize the efficiency of the health care system by encouraging hospitals to specialize in specific services, avoiding duplication within the region. On the Belgian side, in 2010 public authorities set up the

Observatoire pour la mobilité des patients [Observatory for patient mobility] in order to collect precise data about cross-border flows and their costs for the Belgian health care system. These initiatives illustrate the authorities' efforts to create transparency on cross-border patient mobility.

The most important example is the 2005 framework agreement between France and Belgium (see Box 4.1), which national authorities created in an attempt to gain control over and provide a framework for the local and regional collaborations in the border regions. Despite the attempts of public authorities to supervise the collaboration, however, local stakeholders found support in a strong actor – the EU – which creates tools used by field actors to bypass national authorities.

Conclusion

If the ZOAST Ardennes agreement functions successfully, it is because all the actors directly involved have a stake in collaborating and making the cross-border system work. Some of these incentives were easy to understand, but others were more complex.

Although the findings are not necessarily directly relevant to other collaborations at the French–Belgian border, where the volumes of patient flows are much lower and more evenly balanced, several of the mechanisms and stakeholder drivers analysed in this chapter apply to other cooperation initiatives (see, for example, Glinos et al., 2006). Through the collaboration, health care providers and insurers on both sides of the border have striven to position themselves strategically in a health care market they expect to become increasingly international. This may explain the attempts of actors to acquire and retain leadership in their domains.

Insurers and hospitals want to improve their ability to deal with cross-border files, while physicians use the collaboration to expand their reputations. Public authorities try to implement tools to maintain control over local actors' practices, while the EU funds local initiatives designed and implemented by field actors who make creative use of existing frameworks: this weakens the position of national authorities, who risk losing control. Initiatives originally set up as pilot studies or experiments can become established systems without going through proper assessments or political decision-making channels. Field actors feel comfortable setting up agreements and find practical solutions even if these are not in accordance with legal frameworks. The EU offers an opportunity to legitimize cross-border cooperation.

The collaboration is undoubtedly necessary since it guarantees access for (mainly French) patients to nearby health care services. Organizational efforts make the collaboration function and facilitate access to care. On the Belgian side, however, although no specific initiatives were found to prioritize French patients, the fact that high inflows impede domestic patients' access to certain services requires particular attention.

Acknowledgements

We would like to thank all our interviewees for taking the time to speak frankly to us. We are also very grateful to Pascal Garel, Christian Horemans and Chris Segaert for their valuable feedback on earlier versions of this chapter. We extend our gratitude to Claire Albano for her contribution in coding the interviews during her internship at the Observatoire social européen and to Renaud Smoes for drafting the maps.

References

ARH de Champagne-Ardenne (2006). *Schema régional d'organization sanitaire de Champagne-Ardenne.* Châlons-en-Champagne, L'agence régionale d'hospitalization de Champagne-Ardenne (www.champagne-ardenne.pref. gouv.fr/index.php/sgar_gb/media/files/publications/recueil_des_actes_ administratifs/annee_2006, accessed 17 June 2013).

ASMUP 08 (2008). Les soins transfrontaliers: la convention ZOAST Ardennes [web site]. Givet, Association Soins Médicaux Usagers de la Pointe (www.asmup08.fr/pages/les-soins-transfrontaliers-comment-ca-marche/, accessed 17 June 2013).

Glinos IA, Baeten R (2006). *A literature review of cross-border patient mobility in the European Union.* Brussels, Observatoire social européen (www.ose.be/files/publication/health/WP12_lit_review_final.pdf, accessed 17 June 2013).

Glinos IA, Baeten R, Boffin N (2006). Cross-border contracted care in Belgian hospitals. In: Rosenmöller M, McKee M, Baeten R, eds. *Patient mobility in the European Union: learning from experience.* Copenhagen, WHO Regional Office for Europe: 97–118 (www.euro.who.int/__data/assets/ pdf_file/0005/98420/Patient_Mobility.pdf, accessed 14 June 2013).

Harant P (2006). Hospital cooperation across French borders. In: Rosenmöller M, McKee M, Baeten R, eds. *Patient mobility in the European Union: learning from experience.* Copenhagen, WHO Regional Office for Europe: 157–77 (www.euro.who.int/__data/assets/pdf_file/0005/98420/ Patient_Mobility.pdf, accessed 17 June 2013).

INSEE (2010). *Densité des professionnels de santé en Champagne-Ardenne.* Paris, Institut national de la statistique et des études économiques (www.insee.fr/fr/themes/document.asp?reg_id=13&ref_id=15025, accessed 12 July 2012).

INSEE (2012). *Les unités urbaines des Ardennes: la population des territoires de Champagne-Ardenne au 1er janvier 2009.* Paris, Institut national de la statistique et des études économiques (Insee dossier 35 – January 2012; www.insee.fr/fr/themes/document.asp?reg_id=13&ref_id=18222&page=insee_dossier/territoire_rp_2009/rp_2009_uurb_ard.htm, accessed 12 July 2012).

MOT (2012). L'influence croissante de la construction européenne sur les systèmes de santé [web site]. Paris, Mission opérationelle transfrontalière (www.espaces-transfrontaliers.org/theme.php?theme=Sant%E9&idtheme=20&lien=theme/theme_sante.html#experiences, accessed 18 June 2013).

OFBS (2013). Zone organisée d'acces aux soins transfrontaliers [online presentation]. Villeneuve d'Ascq, Observatoire Franco-Belge de la Santé (www.ofbs.eu/acces-aux-soins-transfrontaliers-f-b-2013.html, accessed 6 September 2013).

Annex 4.1 Interviews conducted

Number	Date	Interviewee(s)	Institution
Interview 1	13 October 2010	Manager	Belgian sickness fund
Interview 2	25 February 2011	Manager	Belgian sickness fund
Interview 3	3 May 2011	Manager	Belgian hospital
Interview 4	17 May 2011	Manager	Belgian hospital
Interview 5	1 June 2011	Two managers	Belgian hospital
Interview 6	1 June 2011	Two managers	Belgian hospital
Interview 7	10 June 2011	Three managers	Belgian sickness fund and polyclinics
Interview 8	21 June 2011	Two managers	French SHI fund and VHI fund
Interview 9	29 June 2011	Two managers	French regional health authority
Interview 10	3 October 2011	Two specialists	Belgian hospital
Interview 11	12 October 2011	Health professional	French public primary care service
Interview 12	14 October 2011	Civil servant	NIHDI (Belgium)

Chapter 5

Radiotherapy across the border: treating Danish patients in Flensburg Malteser hospital (Germany–Denmark)

Uta Augustin, Dimitra Panteli and Reinhard Busse

Introduction

According to WHO, "cancer is a leading cause of death worldwide" (WHO, 2011). Indeed, incidence of malignant neoplasms in Denmark has risen significantly in recent decades (National Board of Health, 2005; 2010), increasing by almost 22% between 1998 and 2008 (Fig. 5.1).

Fig. 5.1. *Incidence of malignant neoplasms in Denmark and selected comparators, 1998–2008*

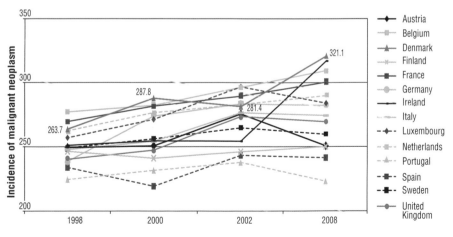

Source: OECD, 2012a.
Note: International Classification of Diseases, tenth revision: C00–C97; no data available for 2004 and 2006; selection criteria for comparators: data available for 1998, 2000, 2002 and 2008.

Cancer treatment capacities, however, were limited during this period, especially for radiotherapy (Interview 1). Until 2006 only six hospitals in Denmark had a radiotherapy department: those at Aalborg, Aarhus, Copenhagen (two hospitals),

Odense and Vejle (both in the Region of Southern Denmark administrative region, 150 km and 110 km from the Danish–German border respectively) (Map 5.1).

Map 5.1. *Geographic distribution of radiotherapy departments and other relevant cities in Denmark and Germany*

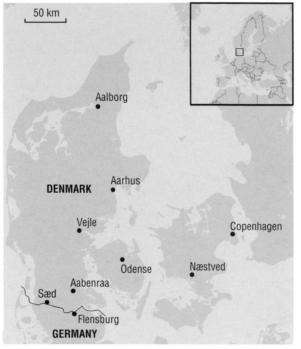

- Aalborg, Aarhus, Copenhagen, Næstved (since 2006), Odense, Vejle: Danish hospitals with a radiotherapy department

- Aabenraa: potential location for a new positron emission tomography–computerized tomography (PET–CT) scanner

- Sæd: residence of the first Danish patient treated in Flensburg

- Flensburg (Malteser St Franziskus Hospital): German hospital cooperating on treatment of Danish patients

Source: Authors' own compilation.

Centralization of highly specialized care and a trend towards fewer but larger hospitals may explain these limited capacities (Strandberg-Larsen et al., 2007). Furthermore, the technical equipment available was partly outdated (National Board of Health, 2005). As a result, cancer patients in Denmark faced both long waiting (Interview 2) and travelling times (Interview 1). As shown by the "HealthACCESS" project (Busse et al., 2006), organizational and geographical issues are the most common obstacles to access to health care, but there is evidence that these can be overcome by cross-border collaborations (Legido-Quigley et al., 2012).

One example of cross-border health care cooperation aiming to alleviate such access problems exists at the German–Danish border region, where the German Malteser St Franziskus Hospital in Flensburg and the Region of Southern Denmark collaborate to provide radiotherapy for Danish cancer patients. This chapter aims to investigate the inception and development, underlying formal regulations and stakeholder incentives involved in this project and to explore its potential for the future.

Methodology

The collaboration was studied using both primary (expert interviews) and secondary (desk research) data. For the latter, the databases Medline and KOBV (Cooperative Library Network Berlin-Brandenburg, a national library database) were used. As a result of the limited number of publications, grey literature such as press releases and lecture notes was included in a second stage. Subsequently semi-structured telephone interviews were carried out. For this purpose, relevant stakeholders of the collaboration (Box 5.1; see Annex 5.1 for interview details) were identified and contacted according to the patient–provider–payer triangle.

Box 5.1. *Institutions contacted and interviewed*

- Aarhus University Hospital
- Cancer Society of Schleswig-Holstein
- Danish Cancer Society (Kraeftens Bekaempelse)
- **Federal State of Schleswig-Holstein – Ministry of Social Affairs, Health, Family and Equality**
- German Cancer Aid
- **Malteser St Franziskus Hospital in Flensburg**
- Ministry of Interior and Health in Denmark
- National Board of Health in Denmark
- Odense University Hospital
- **Region of Southern Denmark**
- **Regional office of the Southern Jutland-Schleswig Region[1]**
- **Southern Jutland Hospital (Sygehus Sønderjylland)**

Note: bold text used for institutions interviewed.

Given the impossibility of contacting Danish cancer patients directly, the Danish Cancer Society was chosen to provide insight into the patient perspective. Managers and the chief physician of the radiation therapy department of Malteser St Franziskus Hospital in Flensburg offered health care provider perspectives. The Region of Southern Denmark also referred researchers to

---

1　The Southern Jutland-Schleswig Region was founded in 1997 to strengthen the shared Danish and German border region and to turn disadvantages caused by geographical or structural weaknesses into advantages through, for example, several collaborative projects (Southern Jutland-Schleswig Region, 2012).

Southern Jutland Hospital, where a representative of the management as well as the chief physician of the oncological department agreed to participate. As well as the local Danish authorities, secondary data analysis revealed that financial support came from the Federal State of Schleswig-Holstein; the authors also contacted a member of staff at this authority, who in turn arranged contact with the Ministry of Social Affairs, Health, Family and Equality. To ensure quality, the authors asked all interviewees to comment on and verify the chapter.

The following sections reflect findings from both data selection approaches to illustrate the characteristics of the collaboration as well as the incentives for its stakeholders.

Context and development of the collaboration

The Danish health care system – a brief overview

Denmark has historically had a decentralized health care system, with responsibilities for primary and secondary care devolved to the national, regional and municipal levels (Olejaz et al., 2012). In 2007 the government introduced a structural reform to define new local and regional authorities. Denmark's 14 counties were abolished and replaced by five regions, and its 271 municipalities were reduced to 98 (Ministry of Interior and Health, 2005). This reorganization also entailed a reallocation of health care responsibilities (Olejaz et al., 2012; Fig. 5.2).

The regions play an important role in providing health care to Denmark's citizens. One of their main activities is securing hospital services (Ministry of Health and Prevention, 2008). Their financial resources consist of a combination of block grants (around 86% in 2011) and activity-related subsidies (around 14% in 2011) from national government and the municipalities (Olejaz et al., 2012). Access to hospital and specialist care is guided by general practitioners (GPs) (Ministry of Health and Prevention, 2008). Unlike in Germany, specialists in Denmark are mostly employed directly by hospitals, which have both inpatient and outpatient clinics (Olejaz et al., 2012). In case of suspicion of cancer, GPs refer patients to a hospital with an oncological department. GPs initially had to refer cancer patients to a public hospital within their county, but a waiting time guarantee (of two months until treatment)[2] introduced in 1999 ensured patient access to

---

2 The 1999 waiting time guarantee applied to 12 life-threatening diseases (including cancer). A general waiting time guarantee was implemented in 2002.

treatment by enabling a free choice of hospital, including hospitals in other counties, private hospitals and hospitals abroad (Østergren et al., 2008; Olejaz et al., 2012). The counties were thereby obliged to set up bilateral agreements for patient referrals (Ministry of Health and Prevention, 2008). In 2007, the waiting time guarantee was reduced to one month. The National Board of Health, however, has to approve treatment administered abroad (Olejaz et al., 2012).

Fig. 5.2. *Danish statutory health care responsibilities at national, regional and municipal levels*

State
- Specialty planning
- Systematic follow-up on quality, efficiency and information technology usage

Regions	**Municipalities**
• Hospitals	• Preventive treatment, care and
• Psychiatry	rehabilitation that do not take place during
• Health insurance (GPs, specialists	hospitalization; special dental care
and reimbursement for medication)	• Home care
	• Treatment of alcohol and drug abuse

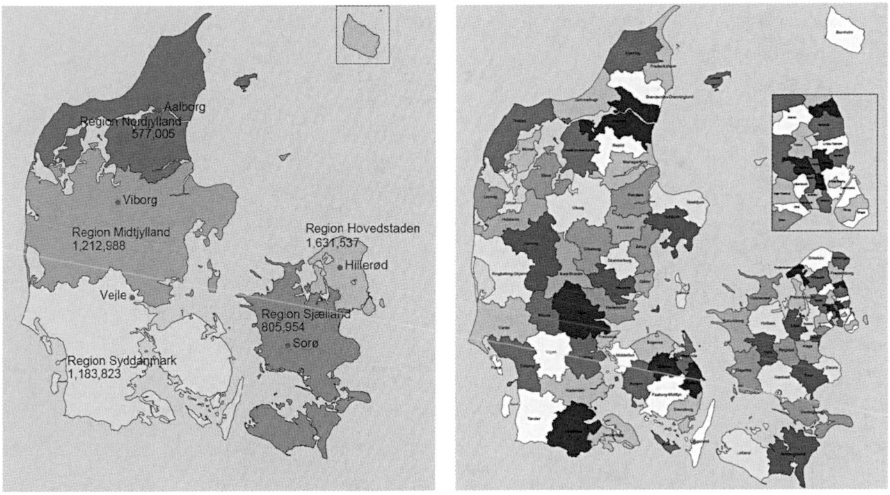

Source: Authors' compilation based on Ministry of Interior and Health, 2006.

Evolution of the collaboration

In November 1997, a Danish cancer patient living in Sæd, close to the German–Danish border, heard about the highly specialized radiotherapy department at the German Malteser St Franziskus Hospital in Flensburg (Brodersen, 2011; Deitmaring, 2008). He was registered to receive radiotherapy in Aarhus, 200 km from his home (see Map 5.1), which would entail travelling 400 km daily for seven weeks. Flensburg, on the other hand, was only 40 km away. The patient worked in retail, so local treatment would enable him to maintain his business, and language was not an issue since he spoke German. He therefore contacted the German hospital and asked to receive the necessary radiotherapy there (Brodersen and Deitmaring, unpublished data, 11 April 2012). This initiated the now well-established cross-border collaboration between Malteser St Franziskus Hospital and the Region of Southern Denmark.

Following his initial request, the patient contacted the public health office of the former County of Southern Jutland (part of the Region of Southern Denmark since 2007) to clarify issues of financing. As a result, the county medical officer visited the German hospital three days later and explained Denmark's general problems regarding the provision of radiotherapy (Brodersen, 2000).

In February 1998, Malteser St Franziskus Hospital contacted the information office of the Southern Jutland-Schleswig Region to initiate discussion of the possibilities of cross-border radiotherapy for Danish cancer patients and to identify relevant contacts in Denmark. Later that same year, after numerous consultations between stakeholders regarding the procedures and comparability of radiotherapy, the hospital and the former County of Southern Jutland signed an initial agreement for provision of services (Interview 1; Brodersen, 2000; Deitmaring, 2008). The agreement included a maximum treatment volume of 100 Danish patients per year and the hospital's obligation to treat in accordance with Danish guidelines (Deitmaring, 2008). Cancer patients in the south of Denmark were thus able to choose between a Danish hospital and the Flensburg Malteser hospital (Interview 2). The National Board of Health also signed a basic contract with Malteser St Franziskus Hospital (Interview 2) giving the hospital permission to treat Danish patients.

Despite the 1999 waiting time guarantee, the issue of long and repeated travel persisted for many cancer patients within Denmark because of the geographical location and scarcity of hospitals with oncological departments, as well as the need for multiple radiotherapy sessions depending on the type and stage of the tumour (Interview 1). In 2001, therefore, the Region of Southern Denmark and Malteser St Franziskus Hospital signed a formal contract including a wider range of indications (curative and palliative treatment of various types of cancer, primarily breast cancer), an increased maximum patient volume (300 per year) and co-financing of a second linear accelerator (see section on "Organization and financing") (Interview 2; Deitmaring, 2008; Brodersen and Deitmaring, unpublished data, 11 April 2012).

In parallel, authorities made great efforts to improve the capacity and equipment of Danish radiotherapy departments. From 1997 to 2002 the number of accelerators increased by 46% (National Board of Health, 2004) but in total capacities remained low. As a result, the National Board of Health developed recommendations for regions to implement on prevention, diagnosis and treatment pathways, rehabilitation and palliative care, published in 2005 within the *National Cancer Plan II* (National Board of Health, 2005).

In 2006, the Region of Southern Denmark decided to extend the contract with Malteser St Franziskus Hospital for five years and expand it to referral regions nationally to make the treatment options available to patients from all over Denmark (Interview 2; Deitmaring, 2008). Furthermore, treatment in Flensburg attained the status of a domestic capacity (Ministry of Interior and Health, 2007). The Region extended the contract once again in November 2011 for another period of five years (until 31 December 2016) – signatories were the Regional Council of Southern Denmark and Regional Director of Health Affairs (Interview 8), as well as Malteser St Franziskus Hospital (Brodersen and Deitmaring, unpublished data, 11 April 2012).

Organization and financing

Once Danish cancer patients – primarily patients in the Region of Southern Denmark – receive confirmation of an indication for radiotherapy, they have the choice of receiving treatment in Flensburg or at a Danish hospital. If they opt for the former, the referring hospital contacts the Malteser hospital to check capacity for treatment and submits all necessary documents such as examination and surgery records (Interviews 1 and 2). Upon completion of treatment, the Flensburg Malteser hospital provides a corresponding final report to the referring hospital, including diagnosis and tumour stage as well as a record of radiotherapy performed (Interview 1). All documents are in the national language of the issuing hospital to avoid liability issues, although the majority of personnel speak Danish and German on both sides of the border (Interview 1). Radiation treatment in Flensburg is primarily an ambulatory service (depending on the type and stage of the tumour) and follow-up takes place in Denmark, with the exception of recurrences requiring further radiotherapy (Interview 2).

By 2011 more than 2000 Danish cancer patients had undergone radiotherapy in Malteser St Franziskus Hospital (Interview 2). The annual number of Danish patients treated in Flensburg increased steadily until 2007 (Fig. 5.3) but has fluctuated since, probably as a result of increased capacities in Denmark, according to estimates from the Danish Ministry of Interior and Health (2007).

Fig. 5.3. *Danish patients treated in Malteser St Franziskus Hospital, 1998–2010*

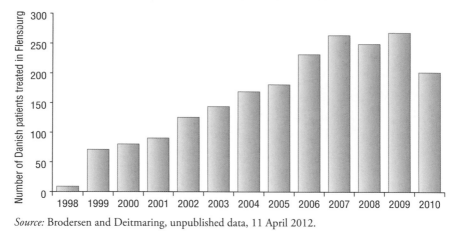

Source: Brodersen and Deitmaring, unpublished data, 11 April 2012.

The treatment follows Danish clinical and quality guidelines (Interview 1). For instance, breast cancer patients normally receive 25–33 radiation sessions over a period of five to seven weeks as determined by Danish treatment protocol (Brodersen and Deitmaring, unpublished data, 11 April 2012). To facilitate knowledge transfer, the chief physician of Malteser St Franziskus Hospital participates in Danish specialist societies (Interviews 1 and 8). The hospital is also included in Danish quality studies (Interview 2) and was until recently the only foreign hospital listed in the Danish hospital plan (Interview 5; Brodersen, 2008). Nevertheless, German requirements such as the Radiation Protection Ordinance (Federal Office for Radiation Protection, 2012) are also mandatory (Interview 5). Danish physicians from related fields in their turn are members of the "Tumorzentrum Flensburg", an interdisciplinary cooperation network between physicians of the Southern Jutland-Schleswig Region, the city of Flensburg and the counties of Schleswig-Flensburg and Northern Friesland, led by the chief physician of Malteser St Franziskus Hospital's radiotherapy department (Interview 1; Deitmaring, 2008).

Financing and reimbursement of services are two crucial issues in cross-border health care. In 2001, Malteser St Franziskus Hospital had to consider expansion of its facilities, personnel and technical equipment, since the radiotherapy department was gradually reaching capacity limits (Interview 1). The hospital received subsidies from the Federal State of Schleswig-Holstein amounting to €2.35 million (Eick, 2000) and Denmark agreed to provide financial support (€500 000) for a new linear accelerator (radiotherapy device) (Interview 2). Further expansion and the purchase of a third linear accelerator became necessary in subsequent years. This expansion and modernization was financed by the hospital investing €750 000 of stakeholder equity (Mumm, 2011), local subsidies for hospital investment financing foreseen in the state hospital plan and national subsidies (under the second economic stimulus programme) to a total amount of €3 million (Ministry of Social Affairs, Health, Family and Equality, 2012).

The Region of Southern Denmark pays for radiotherapy for Danish cancer patients in Flensburg on a fee-for-service basis: prices are based on the German medical fee schedule for care outside the statutory health insurance scheme (GOÄ – Gebührenordnung für Ärzte) (Interview 2). In contrast, radiotherapy in Danish hospitals is reimbursed using a diagnosis-related group (DRG) rate. Glinos and Baeten (2006) investigated the collaboration and found that prices in German hospitals are 10% lower than the Danish DRG rates; the Region of Southern Denmark confirmed this, but price differences seem to be marginal (Interview 8).

Stakeholder incentives

One of the main aims of this study was to explore stakeholders' reasons for contributing to the collaboration. All interviewees pointed out that the principal motivation is the benefit to Danish patients: not only can patients receive their radiotherapy much more promptly (Interview 5) but their travelling time from the Region of Southern Denmark is substantially reduced (Interview 2). Since Denmark greatly expanded its capacities (Fig. 5.4), the collaboration is in theory no longer necessary (Interviews 2 and 6). Nevertheless, the benefit of shorter travelling times remains for cancer patients in the Region of Southern Denmark (Interviews 2 and 8).

Fig. 5.4. *Development of radiotherapy equipment in Denmark, 2000–2011*

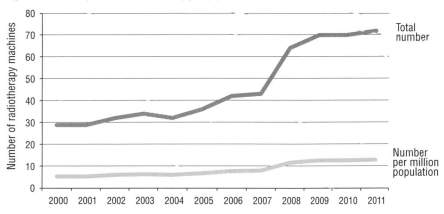

Source: OECD, 2012b.
Note: Data until 2007 for radiation absorbed dose (RAD) units include only linear accelerators. From 2008, all types are included (machines used for treatment with x-rays or radionuclide: linear accelerators, Cobalt-60 units, Caesium-137 therapy units, low to orthovoltage x-ray units, high dose and low dose rate brachytherapy units and conventional brachytherapy units).

The management of Malteser St Franziskus Hospital pointed out that – in light of the ideological model of the Order of Malta to which it belongs,[3] combined with the historical background of the two regions – this cross-border collaboration fosters an even stronger bond between the two countries in the border region (Interview 2). In addition, physicians in Flensburg need to have a good understanding of the health systems, quality standards and treatment guidelines of both countries, and Danish and German specialists collaborate within specialist societies; this ensures better treatment quality for both German and Danish patients (Interviews 1 and 2), which interviewees considered one of the main advantages. Furthermore, the project fits into the hospital's strategic plan, since radiotherapy is one of its two specialties: it thus offers a competitive advantage, but in a national rather than regional or local context due to both the distribution of specialties among Flensburg hospitals (Interview 2) and the substantial distance to other radiotherapy departments in the Federal State of Schleswig-Holstein. The head of the health care department of the Ministry of Social Affairs, Health, Family and Equality of Schleswig-Holstein (Interview 5) commented that the collaboration is advantageous to the hospital's reputation. There are also financial incentives for Malteser St Franziskus Hospital. Considering that the radiotherapy department was set up in 1982, the collaboration has contributed to its continuation, maintenance, expansion and modernization (Interviews 1 and 2). Furthermore, proximity to the border makes Denmark an additional market for the hospital: Danish revenues are supplementary to the nationally assigned budget (Interview 2).

The Federal State of Schleswig-Holstein has also subsidized the collaboration for a number of reasons. From the perspective of the secretariat and information office for cooperation in the border region of Southern Jutland-Schleswig, the fact that the collaboration contributes to an efficient self-financing hospital is an incentive for the Federal State (Interview 4). Besides, Denmark has long been an important partner for Schleswig-Holstein: many mutual projects are in place in economic and cultural fields (Interview 5). Cooperation in the field of health care, however, has faced restrictions from both the different systems in place and uncertainty regarding reimbursement for services obtained abroad (Interview 5). The project thus pioneers health care-related cross-border collaboration (Interview 2). It also fits well within the Federal State's local planning: infrastructural weakness within the region requires collaborations that ensure provision and guarantee high-quality medical services (Interview 3).

---

3   A Christian order whose inspiring principle is to assist the poor and suffering, represented worldwide through various humanitarian institutions, particularly in the social and medical domain (Order of Malta, 2012).

Denmark's incentives to collaborate were strongest when its national radiotherapy capacities were still insufficient, since it gave Danish cancer patients the option to receive treatment much earlier and closer to home (Interviews 6 and 8). The expansion of radiotherapy capacities in recent years (Table 5.1) removed the incentive of shorter waiting times (Interviews 6 and 8). Nevertheless, the option of receiving radiotherapy in Flensburg remains important for proximity reasons, particularly for patients living in the border region (Interview 2).

Table 5.1. *Danish radiotherapy capacity and demand (estimated), 2007–2009*

	Capacity per year		
Institution	**2007**	**2008**	**2009**
Aalborg	22 000	25 400	26 400
Aarhus	37 699	46 698	60 651
Flensburg	7 365	8 220	8 220
Herlev, Copenhagen	47 210	54 654	57 000
Næstved (since 2006)	0	6 670	10 070
Odense	29 331	36 667	45 000
Rigshospitalet, Copenhagen	57 300	67 830	66 930
Vejle	19 750	25 642	31 000
Total estimated capacity	**220 655**	**271 781**	**305 271**
Total estimated demand	**265 331**	**284 247**	**305 590**
Difference	**−44 676**	**−12 466**	**−319**

Source: Ministry of Interior and Health, 2007.

Despite the extension of the contract in November 2011 (Interview 2), the combination of increased capacities (Interview 6) and the simultaneous flow of Danish finances into Germany raises questions about the incentives of the Region of Southern Denmark to maintain the collaboration (Interviews 1 and 5). One important aspect is the high level of patient satisfaction, and the continuing advantage of a local treatment option plays an essential role (Interview 8). All interviewees emphasized that Danish cancer patients treated at Malteser St Franziskus Hospital are very satisfied with both treatment quality and length of travel time. Given that the corresponding Southern Jutland Hospital is also very satisfied with the cross-border collaboration, it would have been perceived as a regressive step not to renew the contract in 2011 (Interview 8). Nevertheless, there is a need to discuss how to make the beneficial collaboration financially sustainable in times of austerity (Interview 1).

Development of a mutual exchange of medical services with reciprocal reimbursement offers an opportunity to maintain or even expand the collaboration (Interviews 1 and 6). Ambulatory care could, for instance, be a useful starting point: in the Federal State of Schleswig-Holstein it suffers from structural changes in health care provision due to the increasing average age of active physicians (Interview 5). Certain specialized treatments are not available on the German side, even though Malteser St Franziskus Hospital is a maximum care hospital. The Region of Southern Denmark has initiated several discussions concerning fields in which a mutual exchange would make sense (Interview 8). One possibility is positron emission tomography–computed tomography (PET–CT) scanning, for which Germany has a limited indication spectrum and restricted reimbursement by statutory health insurance (Interview 2). While Malteser St Franziskus Hospital has no PET–CT scanner, some Danish hospitals in the Region of Southern Denmark are equipped and shared use could offer a chance to extend the collaboration, with relevant patients sent from Germany to Denmark for diagnosis (Interviews 2 and 5). Given the free choice of provider for German patients, however, this would be of greatest use if available at a hospital near the German–Danish border. Denmark is considering whether to purchase two PET–CT scanners, one of which could be installed in Aabenraa (next to the border: see Map 5.1), or to maintain centralized PET–CT services in Vejle and Odense (Interview 8). Negotiations are also continuing about an expansion of the indications treated in Flensburg: for example, additional treatment of prostate cancer patients (Interview 5).

A bilateral patient exchange is difficult to establish in practice, hampered mostly by the different health care systems (Interview 3), especially the plurality of authorities involved in providing, financing and reimbursing health care services on the German side (Interviews 1 and 2). While in Denmark the regions are primarily responsible for ambulatory and hospital care, structures in Germany are more complex. For instance, the patient's sickness fund must provide authorization for planned hospital treatment abroad to ensure reimbursement (Interview 3). The large number of sickness funds in Germany means that regional representatives of all the funds would need to participate in negotiations in order to agree a bilateral patient exchange: this asymmetry of negotiation partners complicates the issue of treating German patients in Denmark (Interview 1). Although the situation is different in the case of ambulatory care (German patients may seek ambulatory care abroad without prior authorization and services are reimbursed according to national prices) an agreement cannot be forced through because utilization of cross-border services is ultimately a patient's individual decision.

Nevertheless, all interviewees pointed out that a bilateral exchange would be very useful and may in part prove necessary in the future. Joint planning of a regional health infrastructure would be advantageous to all stakeholders

(Interview 1), leading to financial savings related to lower travel costs[4] and the fact that German prices are marginally lower than those of Danish DRGs, which are based on average costs (Interview 8; Glinos and Baeten, 2006). Furthermore, patients could receive high-quality local health care and structural weakness in both regions could be counteracted (Interviews 3 and 5). Interviewees felt that possibilities in border regions stemming from local proximity should be used more efficiently (Interview 1).

Conclusion

This chapter illustrates how cross-border health care collaborations can play an important role in the provision of services to patients living in border regions. It is quite clear, however, that such projects require both engaged initiators and continuing political support in order to overcome differences in health care systems and resulting financing issues.

While initially all stakeholders benefited – patients because of shorter waiting times and travel distances; payers because of timely patient care, reduced travel costs and knowledge exchange; and providers also because of knowledge exchange and additional financial means covering maintenance and expansion expenses – the elimination of the Danish capacity constraint caused new challenges and requirements. The benefit for the Region of Southern Denmark may thus have decreased but the importance of high patient satisfaction thanks to short travel distances remains and is the main reason for maintaining the collaboration. Nevertheless, for the Danish side continuing the collaboration means a flow of finance out of the national health system while capacities in the country remain unused. In times of limited financial resources, considering the possibilities for re-establishing a win–win situation for all parties involved is critical. One option would be to expand the collaboration so that German patients use Danish health care services – a development which remains challenging because of the multiple decision-makers involved on the German side. Although the project was not part of a European funding programme, this might offer another way to simplify and promote the collaboration. Furthermore, joint infrastructure planning could support patients in their decision-making regarding use of cross-border care.

In conclusion, bilateral cross-border health care collaborations can produce substantial added value for patients. They can counteract structural problems, especially in rural peripheral regions, and increase efficiency by avoiding

---

4   In some cases, patients' travel costs are covered (Ministry of Health and Prevention, 2008), such as when the distance between a patient's residence and the hospital exceeds 50 km and transportation costs exceed 60 Danish kroner (about €8) (Region of Southern Denmark, 2011).

redundant structural duplication and through provision of complementary health care services. Ultimately, cross-border collaborations also make an important contribution by fostering the bond between countries and thus enforcing the idea of the European Union.

References

Brodersen HJ (2000). Behandlung dänischer Patienten in der Flensburger Strahlentherapie [web site]. Flensburg, Das Malteser St Franziskus-Hospital (http://hjb-fl.homepage.t-online.de/kliniklp.htm#Hej,%20taler%20du%20dansk, accessed 10 January 2012).

Brodersen HJ (2008). 10 Jahre deutsch-dänische Strahlentherapie in Flensburg [web site]. Flensburg, Das Malteser St Franziskus-Hospital (http://hjb-fl.homepage.t-online.de/ddkstrth.pdf, accessed 10 January 2012).

Brodersen HJ (2011). Das Tumorzentrum stellt sich vor: Eine Einrichtung im Dienste tumorkranker Menschen [web site]. Flensburg, Tumorzentrum Flensburg (www.tumorzentrum-flensburg.de/, accessed 10 January 2012).

Busse R, Wörz M, Foubister T, Mossialos E, Berman P (2006). *Mapping health services access: national and cross-border issues (HealthACCESS). Final report.* Brussels, European Health Management Association (http://ec.europa.eu/health/ph_projects/2003/action1/docs/2003_1_22_frep_en.pdf, accessed 19 June 2013).

Deitmaring K (2008). *Chancen und Risiken der Krankenhäuser bei grenzüberschreitender Gesundheitsversorgung am Beispiel des Malteser Krankenhauses St Franziskus-Hospital.* Flensburg, Malteser St Franziskus-Hospital (www.deutscher-krankenhaustag.de/de/vortraege/pdf/Deitmaring.pdf, accessed 10 January 2012).

Eick J (2000). Modernisierung der Strahlentherapie in Flensburg [web site]. Flensburg, Tumorzentrum Flensburg (http://hjb-fl.homepage.t-online.de/kliniklp.htm#Modernisierung%20der%20Strahlentherapie%20in%20Flensburg, accessed 10 April 2012).

Federal Office for Radiation Protection (2012). *Ordinance on the Protection against Damage and Injuries Caused by Ionizing Radiation (Radiation Protection Ordinance).* Salzgitter, Bundesamt für Strahlenschutz (www.bfs.de/de/bfs/recht/rsh/volltext/A1_Englisch/A1_02_12_StrlSchV.pdf, accessed 21 June 2013).

Glinos IA, Baeten R (2006). *A literature review of cross-border patient mobility in the European Union.* Brussels, Observatoire social européen (www.ose.be/files/publication/health/WP12_lit_review_final.pdf, accessed 10 January 2013).

Legido-Quigley H, Glinos IA, Baeten R, McKee M, Busse R (2012). Analysing arrangements for cross-border mobility of patients in the European Union: a proposal for a framework. *Health Policy* 108(1): 27–36.

Ministry of Health and Prevention (2008). *Health care in Denmark.* Copenhagen, Ministeriet for Sundhed og Forebyggelse (www.im.dk/Aktuelt/ Publikationer/Publikationer/~/media/Filer%20-%20Publikationer_i_pdf/ 2008/UK_Healthcare_in_dk/pdf.ashx, accessed 10 January 2012).

Ministry of Interior and Health (2005). *The local government reform – in brief.* Copenhagen, Indenrigs- og Sundhedsministeriet (www.sm.dk/data/ Lists/Publikationer/Attachments/291/Kommunal_UK_screen.pdf, accessed 10 January 2012).

Ministry of Interior and Health (2007). *Kapacitet på stråleområdet 2007–2009 [Radiotherapy capacity 2007–2009].* Copenhagen, Indenrigs- og Sundhedsministeriet (www.sum.dk/Aktuelt/Nyheder/Tal_og_analyser/2007/ April/Kapacitet_paa_straaleomraadet.aspx, accessed 12 April 2012).

Ministry of Social Affairs, Health, Family and Equality (2012). *Gesundheitsminister Garg: Einweihung eines modernen Linearbeschleunigers im Malteser Krankenhaus St Franziskus-Hospital in Flensburg* [press release]. Kiel, Ministerium für Soziales, Gesundheit, Familie und Gleichstellung (www.schleswig-holstein.de/ArchivSH/PI/MASG/2012/120216_masg_ Flensburg.html, accessed 12 April 2012).

Mumm F (2011). Dritter Linearbeschleuniger am Malteser Krankenhaus St Franziskus-Hospital [web site]. Flensburg, Tumorzentrum Flensburg (http://hjb-fl.homepage.t-online.de/kliniklp.htm#Dritter%20Linearbeschleuniger, accessed 10 January 2012).

National Board of Health (2004). Summary and proposals for focus areas. In: National Board of Health – Danish Centre for Evaluation and Health Technology Assessment. *Evaluation of the Danish National Cancer Action Plan – status and future monitoring.* Copenhagen, Sundhedsstyrelsen: 26–42 (www.sst.dk/publ/Publ2004/kraeft_eva/evaluering_engelsk_resume_.pdf, accessed 14 April 2012).

National Board of Health (2005). *National Cancer Plan II – Denmark.* Copenhagen, Sundhedsstyrelsen (www.sst.dk/publ/Publ2005/PLAN/ kraeftplan2/KraeftplanII_UK/KraeftplanII_UK_med.pdf, accessed 10 January 2012).

National Board of Health (2010). *Det danske sundhedsvæsen i internationalt perspektiv [Danish health care in an international perspective]* Copenhagen, Sundhedsstyrelsen (www.sst.dk/publ/Publ2010/DOKU/OECD/ DKsundhedsv_internationaltpersp.pdf, accessed 19 July 2012).

OECD (2012a). OECD Health Statistics: OECD Health Data: health status [online database]. Paris, Organisation for Economic Co-operation and Development (www.oecd-ilibrary.org/social-issues-migration-health/data/ oecd-health-statistics/oecd-health-data-health-status_data-00540-en, accessed 23 May 2012).

OECD (2012b). OECD Health Statistics: OECD Health Data: health care resources [online database]. Paris, Organisation for Economic Co-operation and Development (www.oecd-ilibrary.org/content/data/ data-00541-en, accessed 23 May 2012).

Olejaz M, Juul Nielsen A, Rudkjøbing A, Okkels Birk H, Krasnik A, Hernández-Quevedo C (2012). Denmark: health system review. *Health Systems in Transition* 14(2): 1–192 (www.euro.who.int/__data/assets/ pdf_file/0004/160519/e96442.pdf, accessed 19 June 2013).

Order of Malta (2012). Mission [web site]. Rome, Order of Malta (www.orderofmalta.int/the-order-and-its-institutions/225/mission/?lang=en, accessed 14 April 2012).

Østergren K, Vrangbæk K, Winblad Ulrika (2008). *Waiting time guarantees in the Scandinavian countries – symbols or reality?* [working paper]. Bergen, Norwegian School of Economics and Business Administration.

Region of Southern Denmark (2011). Facts about the Region of Southern Denmark [web site]. Vejle, Region Syddanmark (www.regionsyddanmark.dk/ wm230808, accessed 10 January 2012).

Southern Jutland-Schleswig Region (2012). Die Kooperation der Region [web site]. Padborg, Southern Jutland-Schleswig Region (www.region.de/ index.php?id=8&L=0, accessed 10 January 2012).

Strandberg-Larsen M, Nielsen MB, Vallgårda S, Krasnik A, Vrangbæk K, Mossialos E (2007). Denmark: health system review. *Health Systems in Transition* 9(6): 1–164 (www.euro.who.int/__data/assets/pdf_file/ 0004/80581/E91190.pdf, accessed 19 June 2013).

WHO (2011). Cancer: fact sheet 297 [web site]. Geneva, World Health Organization (www.who.int/mediacentre/factsheets/fs297/en/index.html, accessed 06 January 2012).

Annex 5.1 Interviews conducted

Number	Date	Interviewee	Institution
Interview 1	13 October 2011	Dr Hans-Jürgen Brodersen, Chief Physician, Radiotherapy Department	Malteser St Franziskus Hospital (Flensburg)
Interview 2	20 October 2011	Klaus Deitmaring, Managing Director	Malteser St Franziskus Hospital (Flensburg)
Interview 3	1 November 2011	Dr Christian Utler, Clinical Director	Malteser St Franziskus Hospital (Flensburg)
Interview 4	17 October 2011	Peter Hansen, Head of the Southern Jutland-Schleswig Regional Office	Southern Jutland-Schleswig Region
Interview 5	7 November 2011	Dr Renée A.J. Buck, Head of Health Care Department	Ministry of Social Affairs, Health, Family and Equality, Schleswig-Holstein
Interview 6	7 November 2011	Søren Aggestrup, MD, DMSc, MPO, Chief Medical Director	Southern Jutland Hospital
Interview 7	7 November 2011	Lene Adrian, MD, Chief Physician, Oncological Department	Southern Jutland Hospital
Interview 8	22 May 2012	Morten Jakobsen, Department of Health, Planning and Development	Region of Southern Denmark

Official projects, grass-roots solutions: the Sami people using cross-border health services in the Teno River valley (Finland–Norway)

Riikka Lämsä, Ilmo Keskimäki and Simo Kokko

Introduction

This chapter focuses on a cross-border health care collaboration in a fringe region of the European Union (EU) between Finland and Norway. The countries have a common border to the north, in a sparsely populated area where distances between inhabitants and service providers are very long. The Sami people, the only indigenous culture in the EU, live in this region: 60–70% of the area's 70 000–100 000 Sami speakers live in Norway and about 10% in Finland.

Finland, Sweden and Norway collaborate in various ways in their adjoining northern sections. This chapter examines the Finnish and Norwegian official and unofficial health care cross-border collaboration in the Teno River valley. The chapter explores the content of the collaboration and highlights the benefits and challenges.

Methodology

The authors based their findings on both desk research and theme interviews. For context, they studied the national and regional agreements underpinning the collaboration and plans of projects for its development, as well as relevant research and other written material on the Sami culture concerning health care and border area collaboration. For a more in-depth understanding of the project they conducted seven interviews between 18 and 28 June 2012; these were mainly in person (one was by telephone) at the interviewees' workplaces or at home (see Annex 6.1 for interview details). They identified central actors in the collaboration as initial interview participants, selecting further interviewees by the snowball sampling method from a wide range: these included local health care administrators and professionals from both sides of the border and representatives of the Sami people.

The interviewees were asked to describe the operation of the cross-border collaboration; to comment on its benefits and disadvantages; to suggest how it could be improved in future; and to identify what kind of threats exist to its continuity. Interviews varied in length from 40 minutes to 2.5 hours and were recorded.

Context and evolution of the collaboration

Geography of the region

The Sami people are an indigenous population inhabiting the Arctic Sápmi area (the region's name in the North Sami dialect), which encompasses parts of far northern Sweden, Norway, Finland and the Kola Peninsula of the Russian Federation. The Sápmi area spans 388 350 km² (about the size of Germany) but is much more sparsely populated, with only 2.3 million inhabitants (versus 82 million in Germany).

This chapter examines the cross-border collaboration between Finland and Norway, which share a lengthy border in the north. The Norwegian region of Finnmark extends across the top of northern Finland, where the northernmost region is commonly known as "Lapland" (Map 6.1). Three Finnish municipalities share the border with Norway (from west to east: Enontekiö, Inari and Utsjoki).

Sami populations and language

Approximately 70 000–100 000 Sami speakers inhabit the four countries: the exact number of Sami people is difficult to determine because censuses and other population data do not record ethnicity, although they record native language. Many Sami speakers have moved away from their original home communities to southern parts of their countries or abroad. Norway has the largest number of Sami people (estimates range between 40 000 and 70 000); Sweden reports an estimated figure of 20 000; in Finland there are about 7500 to 9500 Sami speakers, of whom significant proportions live outside Lapland; and about 2000 Sami people live in the Kola Peninsula of the Russian Federation.

International conventions and the national legislations of Finland, Norway and Sweden guarantee the rights of the Sami people. The Russian Federation's legislation also stipulates some basic rights for indigenous populations.

Map 6.1. *The Sápmi and Teno River valley areas*

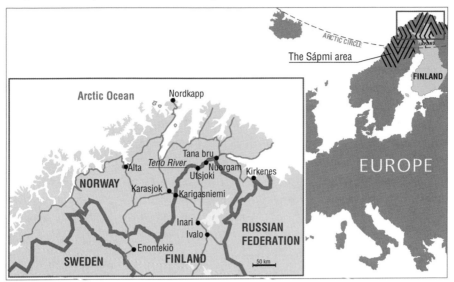

Source: Map graphics SP.

In Finland and Norway, a central legal entitlement of the Sami people is the right to receive public services in the Sami language; this applies to schools, social and health services and other municipal services. This presents a major challenge, at least from the Finnish perspective. The number of Sami speakers in Finland is relatively low and they are spread across a wide and sparsely populated area. There are also few opportunities for young people to stay in their native area as they go through education and seek employment. Furthermore, the Sami language is not a unified one but in fact consists of nine different dialects or languages, and speakers of different variants of Sami do not necessarily understand each other (Näkkäläjärvi and Magga, 2006; Magga, 2010).

As the number of Sami speakers is higher on the Norwegian side of the border, those living in Norway have more opportunity to use their language. The Sami-speaking population is mostly concentrated in the Karasjok–Karigasniemi area of Norway and the municipality of Utsjoki in Finland, where the majority of the 1300 residents list Sami as their native language.

Health care structures

Although both Norway and Finland finance their public services through tax-based funding and deliver them according to residence-based entitlement, their administrative structures are different and somewhat asymmetrical.

In Norway, specialist health care services are the responsibility of the regional health authorities or "helseforetak". The helseforetak for the Finnmark region covers the border with Finland; its administrative centre and main specialist hospital are in Hammerfest. Local municipal authorities are in charge of social services, a range of preventive health services and community nursing. General practitioners (GPs) are, as a rule, private practitioners with a practice based on a contract between the local municipalities (who may organize facilities for practices) and the regional organizations (who channel funding).

On the Finnish side, three municipalities – Enontekiö, Inari and Utsjoki – share a border with Norway. They have their own health centres (Inari's health centre is in the village of Ivalo: see Map 6.1), which are both administrative and service-providing organizations. They offer a wide spectrum of services, including primary care, outpatient clinics and inpatient wards, preventive services and rehabilitation, home nursing and environmental health services. In addition, health centres offer maternity and child health clinics and arrange school health services and population screening.

Cross-border collaboration: history, agreements and plans

No formalities have existed at the border between Finland and Norway since the 1950s, and the international treaties of the European Economic Association (EEA) have actively removed possible obstacles to communication and free movement (Fig. 6.1). As a result, working, shopping and use of all types of everyday services across the border are common. Use of health services has followed the same pattern of multifaceted cross-border interaction to some extent, although both countries base entitlement to "normal" (non-urgent) services on residence status.

The need for cross-border collaboration in the health care sector is clear when considering the geographical settings of both countries' northernmost areas, especially from the Finnish point of view. For example, a resident of the municipality of Utsjoki would need to travel 450 km to reach the nearest operative or obstetric care hospital in Finland at Rovaniemi, or about 700 km to the nearest tertiary-level university hospital at Oulu. Meanwhile, the Karasjok municipality in Norway offers particular specialized health care services "only" 120 km away from Utsjoki (Fig. 6.2).

As a consequence of their location, Finland and Norway have had reciprocal arrangements and formal agreements in the health care and social sectors for many years. In 2004 the prime ministers of both countries launched a joint initiative to map all needs and opportunities for cooperation in public services across the border (Rajoitta pohjoisessa, 2004). Two formal agreements for cross-border collaboration cover the Teno River valley area: an emergency care and a secondary health care agreement.

Fig. 6.1. *The border bridge between Finland and Norway from Utsjoki, Finland*

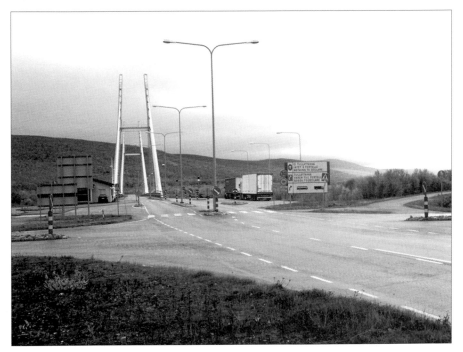

Photograph: Riikka Lämsä.

The national-level agreement on emergency care between the northern parts of Finland, Norway and Sweden came into effect on 1 January 2012.[1] While these countries have collaborated on emergency care since the 1970s, the new agreement formalizes and confirms the cross-border services, ensuring that ambulances and helicopters are available to all countries in emergency situations. The arrangement is crucial to maintaining sufficient capacity and response times for life-threatening cases.

On the Finnish side, municipal health centres are in charge of operating ambulance services – each owns or uses on a contractual basis a number of ambulances calculated to be sufficient for its catchment area. A typical arrangement is to have one vehicle in immediate response readiness and one or more as back-up. Ambulances can, however, easily be in use for hours because of the long distances involved in transporting patients to specialist hospitals. Finland and Norway have agreed procedures for organizing reciprocal ambulance transportation assistance when needed, usually because vehicles are already in use. The same applies to helicopter services. The Finnish helicopter for accident- or illness-related transportation is based at Sodankylä, in the

---

1 Sopimus rajayhteistyöstä ensihoidossa [Agreement on cross-border collaboration in emergency care] (2011). Norbotten County Council, Northern Norway Regional Health Authority, Lapland Hospital District.

Fig 6.2. *Distances around Utsjoki*

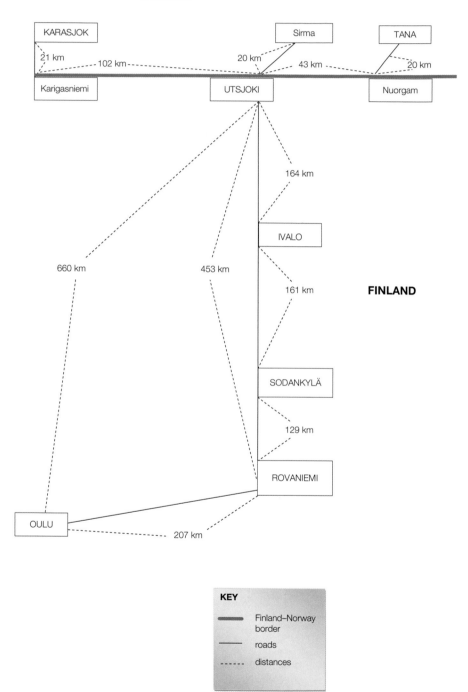

Source: Utsjoki municipality.

middle of Lapland, while the Norwegian service, with several helicopters based at various locations, is more flexible.

In addition, the regional secondary health care authorities of Finland (the Lapland Hospital District in Rovaniemi) and Norway (Finnmark's helseforetak) signed a formal contract on the use of specialist care services across the border in 2007.[2] The services included principally enable Finnish Sami speakers to access care in their native language on the Norwegian side of the border. The agreement also enables the Finnish-speaking population living and working permanently or temporarily in Norway to access Finnish-speaking secondary health care services in Finland, paid for by the Norwegian helseforetak. Use of a patient's mother tongue is particularly important in psychosocial services, where human contact and subtle verbal communication are essential. The agreement covers invoicing practice: the side referring a patient across the border should reimburse all costs to the side providing the service, although in reality cross-border invoicing often proves challenging and local actors find alternative methods, as explained in the section below. Finland has referred obstetric patients to the hospital in Kirkenes and ambulatory patients with cardiology, audiology and psychiatric needs to the physicians' practices in the municipality of Karasjok (see Map 6.1).

The municipality of Utsjoki in Finland and the regional authority of Finnmark in Norway ran closely interlinked collaborative projects in 2005–2007 (Seppänen, 2007). The Finnish side also carried out a new plan to develop social and health services in the Teno River valley in 2010–2012, funded by the Finnish Ministry of Social Affairs and Health (Salminen, unpublished data, 2010). These projects focused on planning, training and information exchange on working methods, practices and colleagues across the border. As well as seeking to guarantee access and availability of services, one strong cross-cutting theme was extending the cultural dimension and ensuring availability of culturally sensitive information regarding the social and health services of Sami people.

Benefits and challenges

Official and unofficial treatment pathways

Existing formal collaboration agreements cover emergency and secondary health care services, especially ambulatory cardiology, audiology, child and adolescent psychiatry and obstetrics. Interviewees reported, however, that many health

---

2   Yhteistyösopimus erikoissairaanhoidosta [Agreement on collaboration in secondary health care] (2007). Lapland Hospital District, Northern Norway Regional Health Authority.

care actors do not have sufficient information about the existence and content of the agreements and do not follow them. For instance, both agreements include details on invoicing the local or regional authority responsible for providing health services to the patient, but Norwegian providers have yet to send invoices to the Finnish health authorities because of the complexities of managing invoices in two different systems as well as the solid Norwegian economy. In some cases the emergency coordination centre in Oulu, 700 km away from Utsjoki, was not aware of the option of requesting a Norwegian ambulance to attend the site of an accident across the border. Occasionally, local physicians in Finland sent patients unofficially straight to Norway – such as for cardiological consultation at Karasjok health centre – without a referral from the Lapland Hospital District, which is the formal procedure according to the secondary health care agreement. Nevertheless, the interviewees felt that the cross-border collaboration was both significant and valuable.

While the official collaboration agreements clarify cross-border treatment pathways and strengthen continuity of care across the border, such safeguards naturally do not exist when patients use unofficial pathways. The municipality of Utsjoki has shown interest in expanding the cross-border collaboration to primary health care services. The motivation is clearly geography: the distance from the village of Nuorgam in Finland to the nearest emergency service unit in the village of Tana in Norway is only 20 km, while on the Finnish side the nearest physician on call is located 200 km away in Ivalo (see Map 6.1 and Fig. 6.2). Since Utsjoki has no more than 1300 residents the collaboration on emergency services at the local health station is not burdening the Norwegian system excessively, but the benefits for Finnish patients in terms of access to services and the savings for the Finnish municipality are potentially significant.

The local Finnish and Norwegian administrations therefore attempted to negotiate an agreement on cross-border collaboration in primary health care services, but this has so far met with no success for two reasons. First, substantial differences exist in the countries' national legislation; second, the need and interest for such collaboration exists mostly on the Finnish side of the border. In consequence, unofficial treatment pathways have emerged: Finnish individuals or families use Norwegian emergency services at the local health station informally "through the back door". According to legislation in both countries all individuals staying in the area even for a short visit are entitled to acute care. Based on this legal provision, Finns use services in Norway for acute but occasionally also for non-acute conditions. Norwegian health service providers have so far permitted this.

The lack of an official collaboration agreement in primary health care causes several challenges for patients, providers and the respective administrations.

Finnish health care providers cannot refer patients to Norway for treatment and private health care providers such as Norwegian GPs cannot advertise their services in Finland. Norwegian physicians are unclear about their responsibilities concerning Finnish patients and patients from Finland do not know their rights to use services across the border. According to the interviewees, however, the most significant challenge concerning unofficial treatment pathways is that they compromise equity among Utsjoki residents. Those patients who are active, have language skills and are self-assured will gain access to cross-border services, while those who follow official rules or who lack knowledge or language skills will not. By and large, the socially disadvantaged are thus worse off in terms of unofficial cross-border health care.

Language issues

The multilingualism of the area is another challenge for cross-border collaboration. Finnish, Norwegian and the dialects of the Sami language differ linguistically to the extent that comprehension across them is impossible. Accordingly, the language issue is present in all cross-border contacts, although inhabitants in the area are commonly multilingual, which assists cooperation. One main aim of the cross-border collaboration is to improve health care services for the Finnish Sami people, but not all residents of the Sápmi area speak Sami. Educated professional inhabitants in particular tend to speak Finnish or Norwegian. In practice this leads to situations where it is essential to know the languages spoken in different offices when intending to use services across the border.

Although the Sami people have a legal right to use their own language in health care services, this has proved a challenge in Finland. For instance, the municipality of Inari has four official languages (Finnish and three Sami dialects), but does not have the financial resources to offer all social and health care services in all four languages, even if it managed to find personnel with the required skills. In fact, challenges to recruiting Sami-speaking qualified staff in Finland make implementation of the law virtually impossible. For instance, no Sami-speaking speech therapist worked in Finland in 2012. Interviewees hoped that municipalities would actively seek and recruit Sami-speaking social and health care professionals for their vacancies, but the bonus of €11 per month for Sami-speaking personnel is understandably far too low an incentive to retain skilful professionals in Finland instead of Norway where salaries are higher. On some occasions, attitudes towards Sami language services have been dismissive because many Sami people can speak Finnish or Norwegian as a second language.

The multilingual context of the cross-border collaboration is complex, although officials, professionals and the population have learned to manage the phenomenon. Collaboration agreements take the issue into account: for instance, the language of referrals and responsibilities for translations are agreed. In addition, Sami-speaking patients have the right to an interpreter hired by the local authority. Since there is a lack of professional interpreters, however, Sami-speaking people commonly visit a doctor with their relative or friend who can speak the physician's language. This is necessarily challenging, especially in psychiatric services. Among health care staff and administrators, simultaneous interpretation would also be a useful way to reduce misunderstandings in cross-border collaboration meetings.

Relationship-led cooperation at grass-roots level

The collaboration between Finland and Norway developed from a response to local needs by professionals at the grass-roots level. The interviewees described this approach as an ideal route to collaboration. For example, physicians working in the area can meet and compare notes on services, customers, problems and needs, and may then jointly agree on treatment pathways, payments, and so on. Local professionals mistrust the top-down approach to cross-border collaboration that only follows administrative statutes from above, but at the same time believe that pressure at the national level could spur on negotiations between local authorities.

Negotiations between local health care actors inevitably face challenges: those based on individual relationships take time and carry risks. If a worker on either side of the border changes, formation of personal contacts and cooperation negotiations have to start afresh. In addition, statutory domestic duties demand most of the health care workers' time and resources, meaning that they cannot prioritize cross-border collaboration. Such cooperation is thus not routine; it is dependent on individual relationships and is vulnerable to changes in health care actors.

Unequal advantages

No official statistics exist on the number of cross-border treatments. There are four main ways Finnish patients gain access to Norwegian health services.

The chief physician of the municipality of Utsjoki refers about one patient a month to Norway for secondary health care service.

A small number of Finnish women use Norwegian obstetric services annually.

Approximately one patient a week uses primary health care services in Norway unofficially.

Some Finnish patients use psychiatric services or services offered by the Sami Crisis and Incest Centre in Norway.

In total, 80–100 Finnish patients use Norwegian health care services per year. The caseload is thus relatively small but far from insignificant in the sparsely populated area. Nevertheless, although official data on patient flows from Norway to Finland in the border region are not available, it is clear that Finnish patients use services in Norway more than Norwegians use services in Finland, so the collaboration is somewhat uneven. Interviewees stated that Norway participates because of solidarity but not financial necessity.

Considering cross-border collaboration and exchanges more broadly, however, and including different sectors and levels, the benefits appear more reciprocal. On the Finnish side the Sami population's entitlement to Sami-speaking services is pressing and cooperation with Norway forms a practical response. The cross-border emergency care and secondary health care agreements are also particularly useful for Finland. In parallel, educated Finns often work on the Norwegian side of the border because of the higher wage level, so Norway receives a qualified workforce – often with Sami language skills – from Finland to its northernmost area, especially in sectors such as health care and construction for which it has difficulty recruiting internally. In the Sevettijärvi area of Inari a public health nurse works two days a week in Norway and three days on the Finnish side of the border, and 50–70 people in Utsjoki commute across the border daily for work (see Map 6.1). Norwegians living in the border area also exploit the lower prices in Finland, purchasing building materials, petrol, alcohol and meat, and using services such as hairdressers and car mechanics across the border.

While Finland currently has little to offer Norway in the health care sector, other fields may offer exchanges for the future. Sectors such as waste management, fire and rescue and schools could set up or improve cooperation, and new collaboration partners might join from outside the public sector (Rajoitta pohjoisessa, 2004).

Health care system differences

Differences between the Norwegian and Finnish health care systems also complicate matters. First, there can be difficulties in finding negotiation partners for cross-border collaboration, even where the will to create an agreement exists, because power and responsibility are located at different levels so that it can be tricky to identify the appropriate actor. Regional or subregional officials do not regard municipal managers as potential negotiators and the national central administration level is not interested in such local activity. In the worst cases the negotiation process does not even start because of a lack of suitable negotiation partners.

The countries' different health care administrative systems cause problems for invoicing. For instance, at the primary care level Norwegian GPs working as private practitioners may find that sending invoices to Finnish municipalities, which should pay all costs, is too complicated. They therefore prefer to refer to Finnish patients as Norwegian and invoice the Norwegian system.

Differences in administration between the countries also complicate the work of health care staff working on both sides of the border. As in the case of the public health nurse working in Finland and Norway, in practice they operate in two different systems and need to change their practices – such as the language used for patient records – when they cross the border. That kind of action requires a specialist level of expertise.

Finally, patients may confront difficulties when using services across the border. Within strictly specified services, such as a cardiologist's ambulatory consultation, the collaboration functions well; however, if the patient's needs require the involvement of many different health care services and actors, administrative and structural differences in the health care systems complicate the situation. For instance, the concept of sick leave is legally different in Norway and Finland. Patients using services across the border also reported difficulties in receiving reimbursements for eligible travel benefits or rehabilitation grants from the national social insurance system.

Traditions of the Sami people

Some interviewees mentioned that traditional Sami ways of life may not contribute to the official collaboration between Finland and Norway. National borders are more or less irrelevant for local Sami people: they have always fished, visited family and married on both sides of the border. In a culture where such practices are usually unofficial, the bureaucratic system with its official contracts is not necessarily the one the Sami population wants to follow. In addition, traditional livelihoods such as fishing and reindeer management still have notable symbolic meanings for the Sami people. In these circumstances, collaboration in the health care sector should not be considered a separate issue but just one dimension of the many interactions between Sami people for whom borders are traditionally of little relevance.

Fear that the collaboration will die out

Most interviewees highlighted a number of reasons for concern that the cross-border collaboration might end. Several commented that the number of Sami people in the area is decreasing because young people in both countries tend to migrate elsewhere for work, while at the same time residents without Sami roots are moving to the area. The new inhabitants have fewer social ties across the border or traditional habits of cross-border cooperation, and in consequence the collaboration is becoming more forced and institutionalized.

Local inhabitants are often hesitant to use cross-border services because information about the available services is inadequate. The interviewees believed that local people should receive more effective information.

Another fear originates in the fact that funding for the collaboration comes from temporary project money (the first project in the Utsjoki area ran from 2005 to 2007 and the second from 2010 to 2012). There is a danger that social networks and knowledge about the health care systems of the other country will disappear when the project ends, meaning that actors will have to reconstruct the collaboration from scratch when a new project begins.

Finally, improvement and continuity of the small-scale cross-border collaboration requires truly motivated actors in a situation where large national health care reforms are ongoing in both Norway and Finland.

Conclusion

The aim of the cross-border collaboration in the northernmost areas of Finland and Norway is twofold: to ensure public services for all residents in the sparsely populated area and to offer culturally sensitive services for the Sami population. This chapter illustrates some of the many challenges facing the collaboration, such as differences in administration and health systems, inequality of access to services, temporary financing mechanisms, multilingualism in the area and an imbalance of benefits creating difficulties for improving the collaboration. As a result, local actors often find unofficial and alternative ways to facilitate cross-border health care.

The interviewees hoped, however, that the collaboration would stabilize and expand to other sectors. Official agreements and permanent funding would guarantee its continuity and would ensure equal availability of services for all residents. The collaboration benefits both border region populations, although in different ways, and produces financial savings for both countries. At its best, it also supports daily informal collaboration between Sami people across the border.

References

Magga R (2010). Saamelaisten sosiaali- ja terveyspalvelujen kehittämisen haasteet Suomessa [Challenges to developing social and health policy for the Sami population in Finland]. *Yhteiskuntapolitiikka* [Social Policy], 75(6): 670–8.

Näkkäläjärvi A, Magga R (2006). Saamelaisväestön sosiaali- ja terveyspalvelujen oikeudenmukainen kohdentuminen ja kehittämistarpeet [Equal allocation and challenges for development in social and health services for the Sami population]. In: Teperi J, Vuorenkoski L, Manderbacka K, Ollila E, Keskimäki I, eds. *Riittävät palvelut jokaiselle. Näkökulmia yhdenvertaisuuteen sosiaali- ja terveydenhuollossa [Adequate services for all. Perspectives on equality in social and health care].* Helsinki, STAKES National Research and Development Centre for Health and Welfare: 100–110.

Rajoitta pohjoisessa (2004). *Työryhmäraportti Suomen ja Norjan välisestä yhteistyöstä pohjoisessa [Without borders in the North. Working group report on the collaboration between Finland and northern Norway].* Helsinki, Ministry of the Interior (www.poliisi.fi/intermin/biblio.nsf/ B9C3CB6C0612E022C2256FA20036E912/$file/292004.pdf, accessed 24 June 2013).

Seppänen R (2007). *Utsjoen kunnan ja Norjan lähialueiden sosiaali- ja terveyspalvelujen koordinaatiohanke 2005–2007. Loppuraportti [Project to coordinate social and health services in the municipality of Utsjoki and border areas in Norway. Final report].* Helsinki, Ministry of Social Affairs and Health (www.utsjoki.fi/media/Sosiaali/Rajaton%20Tenonlaakso/ Loppuraportti%20suomeksi.pdf, accessed 24 June 2013).

Annex 6.1 Interviews conducted

Number	Date	Details	Interviewee	Institution
Interview 1	18 June 2012	Face-to-face, 2 hours 30 minutes	Project coordinator	Finnish municipality
Interview 2	19 June 2012	Face-to-face, 1 hour 20 minutes	Finnish physician working in Norway	Norwegian municipality
Interview 3	19 June 2012	Face-to-face, 1 hour 15 minutes	Chief physician	Finnish municipality
Interview 4	20 June 2012	Face-to-face, 58 minutes	Public health nurse working both sides of the border	Finnish municipality
Interview 5	20 June 2012	Face-to-face, 1 hour 5 minutes	Executive director	Sami representative
Interview 6	20 June 2012	Face-to-face, 1 hour 2 minutes	Director of outpatients services	Finnish municipality
Interview 7	28 June 2012	Telephone, 41 minutes	Director of health services	Norwegian municipality

Chapter 7

Local roots, European dreams: evolution of the Maastricht–Aachen University Hospital collaboration (the Netherlands–Germany)

Irene A. Glinos, Nora Doering and Hans Maarse

Introduction

In the border region between the Netherlands and Germany, the Maastricht Universitair Medisch Centrum+ (MUMC+) [Maastricht University Medical Centre][1] and Universitaetsklinikum Aachen (UKA) [Aachen University Hospital] have collaborated since the 1990s, formalizing their exchanges by signing an agreement in 2004. Soon after, they initiated negotiations with the intention of creating a "European University Hospital" (EUH) by merging the two hospitals and building a new joint "centre of excellence". In parallel, medical teams and researchers have been working across the border in various fields. Over the past 20 years the collaboration has evolved in content, scope, intensity and ambition, but by late 2012 it appeared to be at a crossroads.

The aim of this chapter is twofold: first, to examine how cross-border collaboration between the two university hospitals evolved, looking into its location, history, health system context and the content of collaboration; second, to explain why collaboration occurs and who benefits from it. The findings reveal a complex mix of parameters that led UKA and MUMC+ to collaborate, and later to abandon certain collaboration plans. Unlike other examples of cross-border collaboration, that between the two university hospitals is not driven by the need of local patients to access care but rather by the strategic considerations of the two partners. The analysis puts the cross-border collaboration into perspective and proposes to go beyond explanations of geographical isolation to focus on the wider incentives and stakeholders, interests at play and on the vast complexities present when two large organizations, each embedded in its national health system, collaborate. In many respects, the collaboration

---

1   The name "MUMC+" was introduced in 2008. With the exception of the chronology in Box 7.1, for reasons of simplicity this name is used throughout the chapter to refer to the academic hospital in Maastricht, including for events prior to 2008.

between MUMC+ and UKA represents one of the largest-scale and boldest border region health care initiatives attempted in Europe.

Methodology

The authors based their findings on qualitative research combining interviews and desk research. They carried out semi-structured interviews with 16 stakeholders and observers (see Annex 7.1 for interview details) in English, German or Dutch. Interviews took place in person or the telephone: the authors recorded and transcribed seven interviews; summaries were written for the remainder and two interviewees gave written comments on their summaries. Data collection took place between February and April 2012, with a second round of interviews in September 2012. A number of stakeholders were contacted but were not available for interviews (see Annex 7.2).

Desk research and access to networks of experts enabled identification of interview candidates. These included five groups: those working at the two organizations involved with central roles in the collaboration; staff at the organizations with no involvement in the collaboration; external observers; insurers; and potential competitors. The authors structured interviews around the research questions, adapting them to the position and expertise of respondents. They extracted key themes from the data, clustered and reorganized it following initial analysis. Desk research involving literature from within and outside the field of cross-border collaboration, as well as project reports, (contractual) agreements, official documents, press releases and other grey literature complemented the interview data collection.

As a case study based largely on stakeholder interviews, the analysis is biased by the questions asked, by who agreed to be interviewed and by what they were willing to tell. Each perspective is a piece of the puzzle and stakeholders inevitably give their own versions of events. The authors have done their utmost to validate information collected during interviews. Nevertheless, despite repeated and insistent efforts it was not possible to interview as many actors in Germany as in the Netherlands or to access all written material. Given the authors' pre-existing knowledge of the Dutch setting, the chapter at times represents the Dutch perspective. Owing to a coincidence of timing, the research period was one of relative upheaval and uncertainty as to which way the collaboration would go. This may have contributed to some stakeholders' reluctance to agree to an interview and to talk openly and freely about the collaboration.

Context and content of the Maastricht–Aachen collaboration

The border region

Maastricht is the southernmost city of the Netherlands, located in the province of Limburg. South Limburg is a long, narrow strip of land surrounded by borders (Map 7.1). It is relatively remote owing to its position, history and distinct culture, and the area is often called the "appendix" of the Netherlands. MUMC+ is the eighth and newest Dutch university hospital. Limburg's population is 1.1 million of the country's 16 million.

The German city of Aachen lies 30 km from Maastricht, in the state of North Rhine-Westphalia. UKA is the westernmost university hospital in Germany, 1 km from the Dutch border to the west and 3 km from the Belgian border to the south-west. North Rhine-Westphalia has seven university hospitals for a population of almost 18 million, UKA being the newest.

The location of the two hospitals close to their national borders restricts their domestic hinterlands. Moreover, they operate in an environment dense with other hospitals. Within 35 km of MUMC+ are four local Dutch and three local Belgian hospitals (at Sittard, Heerlen, Brunssum and Kerkrade; Tongeren, Genk and Hasselt (Map 7.1)). The university hospitals of Liege and Leuven in Belgium lie only 34 km and 85 km away. On the German side the city of Aachen alone has three hospitals, and several hospitals close to UKA provide some type of cardiovascular care. Cologne, Dusseldorf and Bonn university hospitals are less than 100 km away. The presence of alternative academic hospitals limits the referral radius of MUMC+ and UKA. Dutch-speaking Belgian hospitals, for example, refer patients to Leuven although Maastricht is closer. In the Netherlands, university hospitals have a strong interest in delivering basic care to cross-subsidize the provision of complex treatments, which means, however, that MUMC+ needs a certain volume of basic care to sustain its academic functions (NMa, 2012).

UKA and MUMC+ are located within the Euregio Meuse-Rhine, a particularly active and long-established entity composed of the wider and adjacent border regions of Belgium, Germany and the Netherlands. Created in the 1970s, the Euregio aims to promote cross-border cooperation and regional development and features numerous cross-border agreements involving hospitals, insurers and health authorities (Harant, 2003; Brand et al., 2008).

Map 7.1. *Dutch province of Limburg and surrounding area*

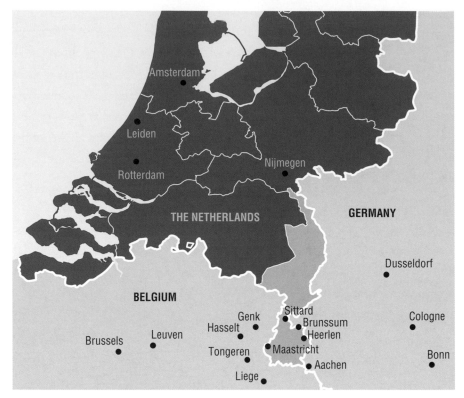

Source: Wikipedia, adapted by the authors.

Evolution of cross-border collaboration

Early days: 1980s to 2004

The executive boards of MUMC+ and UKA met in person in the late 1980s and took the first steps towards collaboration. During the 1990s the two hospitals were partners with the Centre Hospitalier Universitaire Liege (Liege University Hospital) in several cross-border health care projects funded by the successive Interreg i, Interreg ii and Interreg iii programmes,[2] and signed their first contracts involving patient care (Box 7.1; Hermans and den Exter, 1999; empirica GmbH, 2004; Theisen and Heide, 2010). As a result, MUMC+ referred patients to UKA for paediatric heart surgery, positron emission tomography (PET) scans and Gamma Knife operations (Harant, 2003).

Communication between MUMC+ and UKA intensified in the early 2000s, and the hospitals signed a collaboration agreement in June 2004 covering patient

---

2   The partnership was among the first to receive Interreg funding for a health care-related project.

care as well as research (UKA, 2007; Theisen and Heide, 2010). According to this six-page document, the collaboration intended to strengthen and expand highly specialized care and clinical research with the possibility of coordinating resources if financially feasible. The agreement covers aspects of health care provision; training, research and teaching; joint management of medical departments; procedures for staff exchanges; and liability and insurance. It also specifies the drawing up of specific contracts to regulate implementation, such as between collaborating medical departments or to exchange staff.

The agreement provides a flexible framework for collaboration and is not a legally binding document (Interviews 4 and 5). It does not mention any particular medical field, but does give health professional mobility priority over patient mobility.

Gearing up: 2005–2011

Vascular surgery was the first area of active collaboration. MUMC+ and its School for Cardiovascular Diseases were among the leading research centres in the Netherlands. UKA had a strong cardiac department but wished to establish a professorship in vascular surgery, offering the position to the head of surgery and of the cardiovascular centre at MUMC+. In 2005 negotiations resulted in two part-time contracts (40/60%) (Box 7.1). The professor built up the vascular surgery department and UKA installed the chair. The arrangement, in place since October 2005, also suited the MUMC+ leadership, eager to see good intentions materialize: a cross-border vascular centre with a commuting professor was a good way to start the collaboration (Interview 3).

For five years the vascular surgeon was the only physician working at both UKA and MUMC+ (Interview 3). A contract, signed in 2006, allowed the referral of patients for transplants. In 2010, a second professor became head of a department at both hospitals (Box 7.1). One year later, a neurosurgeon from MUMC+ started to operate at UKA (Interview 7).

Meanwhile, the two hospitals' boards discussed how to intensify the collaboration. Plans centred around two projects: the building of a new cross-border cardiovascular "centre of excellence" at the Avantis business park on the border[3] and the merging of the two university hospitals to create the first EUH. The two objectives became intrinsically linked during negotiations and were a compromise between the priorities of the Dutch hospital (to become a European leader in cardiovascular care and research) and the German one (to create one large organization) (Interviews 3, 5 and 10).

---

3   Avantis European Science and Business Park is a cross-border site of 100 hectares, of which 40% is within the territory of the Netherlands and 60% within Germany.

Box 7.1. *Chronology of UKA and MUMC+ and their cross-border collaboration, 1966–2012*

1966   Opening of medical faculty at Aachen University

1974   Opening of medical faculty in Maastricht

1976   Foundation of Rijksuniversiteit Limburg in Maastricht

1976   Creation of Euregio Meuse-Rhine in the border regions of Belgium, Germany and the Netherlands

1985   Inauguration of new university hospital in Aachen

1986   St Annadal Hospital becomes "academisch ziekenhuis Maastricht" (Maastricht Academic Hospital)

1992   First collaboration between the two hospitals and Liege University Hospital in a project co-funded by Interreg i programme

1995   Signing of contracts on the exchange of services in patient care

1996   Official change of name from "Rijksuniversiteit Limburg" to "Universiteit Maastricht" (Maastricht University)

1998   Merger of the three hospitals at Heerlen, Brunssum and Kerkrade effectively begins

2003   New CEO appointed at Maastricht Academic Hospital

2004   (June) Signing of collaboration agreement between UKA and Maastricht Academic Hospital

2005   First health professional starts working at both locations: head of surgery at Maastricht Academic Hospital (since 2000) appointed head of vascular surgery at UKA

2006   Signing of contract for referral of patients for transplants

2008   (January) Maastricht Academic Hospital and Faculty of Health, Medicine and Life Sciences merge to become "MUMC+"

2008   (June) KPMG feasibility study confirming economic rationale of the EUH project

2008   (August) Legal feasibility study by Luther and van Mens Wisselink law firms

2009   (March) GEBERA feasibility study on cross-border cardiovascular centre

2009   (June) Drafting of letter of intent setting out the phases and creation of a joint EUH holding company

2009   (November) New head of cardiology appointed at UKA

2009   Preparation of letter of intent

2010   (June) Head of nuclear medicine at UKA (since 2009) appointed head of nuclear medicine at MUMC+

2011   (January) New CEO appointed at UKA

2012   (January) Official communication calling off building of cross-border cardiovascular centre

2012   (March) UKA renewed part-time contract of head of vascular surgery

Source: authors' compilation based on Harant, 2003; UKA, 2007; Sass and Peeters, 2008; Maastricht UMC+, 2010; Theisen and Heide, 2010; Summum actueel, 2010; Interviews 3 and 10; azM, 2012; Maastricht University, 2009.

In late 2007 the hospitals hired consultancy firm KPMG, Dutch law firm van Mens Wisselink and German law firm Luther to evaluate the feasibility of creating the EUH. The studies concluded that it was financially and legally viable under certain conditions (Theisen and Heide, 2010). The hospitals commissioned GEBERA (a subsidiary of Deloitte) to produce a second feasibility study in 2009, exploring the organizational and economic implications of a common medical strategy and the building of the cardiovascular centre, including a business plan, cost estimation and market analysis. The report came out cautiously in favour of a joint centre based on a spin-off process: the departments of (paediatric) cardiology, (paediatric) cardiac surgery and vascular surgery would be carved out from the parent hospitals and moved to the new centre built at a third location (Avantis). The centre would become a jointly operated subsidiary with economic responsibility for its operations and profits going back to the parent hospitals, according to the letter of intent of June 2009 (Interviews 3 and 5; Bos, 2009).

In parallel, the two law firms negotiated on behalf of the hospitals with authorities in The Hague and Dusseldorf (the capital of North Rhine-Westphalia) until late 2009 (Interview 10). MUMC+ and UKA confirmed their intentions to create a joint EUH holding company and set down the phases of the merger, its composition, management, competences and relationship with the cardiovascular centre in their letter of intent. The document, however, left open the possibility that either partner could decide not to merge.

Development of a business plan for the cardiovascular centre occurred in 2010–2011. Construction was due to start in 2012, with the centre expected to open in early 2015. Estimated total costs were around €200–450 million (Interviews 5, 13 and 14; Bos, 2012; Ittel, 2011).

Change of heart: 2011–2012

Changes were afoot, however. In December 2011 the hospitals took the decision to call off the building plans for the cardiovascular centre at Avantis. According to a press release to employees, the "increasing financial pressures on health care in the Netherlands as well as in Germany, and the uncertainty surrounding future political decisions" meant that the two institutions prioritized internal financial stability and were not prepared to take the risk of costly investments (azM, 2012). The press release stressed that both parties were as committed to cross-border collaboration as before; several interviewees also confirmed this (Interviews 3, 5 and 6). Implicitly, the decision also brought the EUH merger plan to an end.

According to interviewees, UKA and MUMC+ decided to continue to collaborate following a brief reflection period and a new agreement was under negotiation in spring 2012 (Interviews 3, 4 and 5). The hospitals considered redefining the vision of the EUH as a facility assisting cross-border collaboration on a smaller scale and at a slower pace. In mid-2013, however, the authors could not find any sign of a new agreement.

Cross-border collaboration in practice

Table 7.1 gives an overview of the fields and ways in which the two hospitals collaborate. Three points illustrate the logic of sharing and complementarity: the highly specialized character of most medical fields; the prevalence of health professional mobility; and the concentration of patient mobility in low-volume, complex procedures. The overview is not exhaustive as the collaboration adapts in form and content pragmatically according to requirements. Different types of contract allow health professional mobility and patient mobility to alternate as ways of sharing staff, equipment and expertise. One model used is akin to consultancy work: a health professional employed 100% by one hospital sets a proportion of time aside for the partner hospital, which receives an invoice based on hourly rate and number of hours worked. Other health professionals have double employment with part-time contracts at each hospital. UKA and MUMC+ use inter-hospital contracts for patient referrals and for staff secondments, dispatching them to the other hospital on an ad hoc or regular basis.

In certain medical fields the hospitals created plans for joint facilities or so-called "European centres" (on a single location or two sites): for example, in paediatric surgery, neuromuscular diseases, trauma care and transplants. The "Aachen–Maastricht European Vascular Centre", headed by the commuting surgeon, was the first centre abroad accredited by the German Society of Vascular Surgery. German residents can train at MUMC+ and the experience counts towards their degree. The same does not apply for Dutch residents, however, as the equivalent Dutch body does not recognize experience obtained outside the Netherlands (Interview 3; Mols, 2011). One of the most burdensome aspects of day-to-day collaboration is the long bureaucratic procedure of getting health professionals' diplomas recognized, which delays staff exchanges (Interviews 1 and 2).

Table 7.1. *Examples of collaboration activities between UKA and MUMC+, 2005–2011*

Medical field	Description
Patient care: professional mobility	
Paediatric surgery	• Surgeons perform operations together and assist during vacations. • Detachment of MUMC+ surgeon to UKA.
Gastroenterological surgery	• UKA surgeons help MUMC+ in complex bile duct operations. • MUMC+ surgeons help UKA set up laparoscopic hepato-pancreato-biliary programme.

Medical field	Description
Patient care: professional mobility	
Nuclear medicine	• Professor is head of nuclear medicine at UKA (since 2009) and MUMC+ (since 2010).
Cardiovascular care/vascular surgery	• Professor is head of surgery and cardiovascular centre at MUMC+ and head of vascular surgery at UKA, forming the so-called "European Vascular Centre". • Second professor operates at both hospitals. • Hospitals use identical treatment protocols and clinical guidelines.
Neurosurgery	• MUMC+ professor performs deep brain stimulation surgery at UKA where there is no experienced neurosurgeon.
Neurology	• Detachment of UKA specialist in mobility disorders to MUMC+.
Patient care: professional mobility and telemedicine	
Clinical neurophysiology	• MUMC+ professor performs teleneuromonitoring from MUMC+ during vascular operations at UKA, travelling to UKA for complex operations. Five MUMC+ neurophysiologic laboratory technicians travel alternately to UKA when teleneuromonitoring is required. Inter-hospital contract guarantees that one MUMC+ technician is always on call for UKA.
Patient care: patient mobility (with professional mobility)	
Stem cell and liver transplants	• Contract signed in 2006. UKA patients referred to MUMC+ for stem cell transplantations accompanied by UKA specialist. MUMC+ patients referred to UKA for liver and kidney transplantations accompanied by MUMC+ specialist, with pre- and postoperative care at MUMC+.
Cardiac surgery	• MUMC+ patients undergo open heart operations at UKA under MUMC+ rules to optimize capacity.
Trauma care	• MUMC+ trauma department recognized as a member (level 1) of Aachen trauma network.
Plastic surgery	• MUMC+ plastic surgeon occasionally operates on Dutch patients (for breast reconstruction) at UKA because of undercapacity at MUMC+.
Research and education	
Oncology/ radiology	• Project running in 2011–2015 involving MAASTRO clinic, MUMC+, UKA, Liege University Hospital, Maastricht University and Aachen University to set up a proton therapy centre.
Cardiovascular	• Collaboration between School for Cardiovascular Diseases (MUMC+) and Institute for Molecular Cardiovascular Research (UKA).
Neurosciences	• Joint European MSc in Neurosciences, with ERASMUS co-financing (Marie Curie Early Stage Training Site). • Application for "extended visiting professorships" for three MUMC+ professors to teach in Aachen, and three UKA professors to teach in Maastricht.
Nephrology	• Collaboration in research; international course under development.
Various	• Frequent exchanges of PhD students. • Joint research proposals: e.g. Professor at UKA was granted funding for the School for Cardiovascular Diseases (MUMC+) in 2009.

Sources: information made available by MUMC+, adapted by author and complemented by Interviews 1, 2 and 3; Brand et al., 2007; UKA, 2007; Summum actueel, 2010; Ittel, 2011; Doering et al., 2013; Euregio, 2012.

Note: some collaboration activities may have ceased to exist or may never have materialized.

Reasons and incentives for collaboration

A key objective of this study was to understand what drives MUMC+ and UKA to collaborate. The authors identified six sets of reasons from the stakeholder interviews, complementing these findings with information from written sources where necessary.

The need for concentration of expertise

The collaboration uses a strategy of joining forces to become "a leading European medical centre" (Sass and Peeters, 2008); it creates volume, improves quality of care and research and strengthens the hospitals' positions (Interviews 1, 2, 3, 4, 5, 10 and 13). Specialization and "excellence" are necessary to compete at national and European levels: the "ambition is to be in the top three of Europe, not only in research but also in treatment of patients in certain fields – not every field but certain ones" (Interview 5). For complex and/or low-volume procedures, performing (for example) 20 extra deep brain stimulation surgeries or transplants per year makes a difference. Both hospitals previously had difficulty reaching minimum levels for transplants (Brand et al., 2007). Moreover, collaboration avoids duplication and increases efficiency (for example, with joint investment in a particle accelerator or sharing salary expenses for senior medical staff) (Interviews 1, 3, 4, 5 and 10).

Concentration is a priority of recent Dutch reforms, encouraging hospitals to improve quality and cut costs (see, for example, PRV-Limburg, 2010). Specialization is crucial for "strategic positioning" as hospitals compete to reach volume criteria (Interviews 1 and 2) and the expectation is that health insurers will intensify selective contracting from 2013. Collaboration networks are also appearing, as in the west of the Netherlands between university hospitals such as Amsterdam, Rotterdam and Leiden (Interview 3). In the German hospital sector, the number of facilities increases competition, while quality assurance regulations define activity thresholds (Interview 2). Volume requirements were introduced in 2002 for elective care such as kidney and liver transplants (Palm et al., 2013). MUMC+ sends patients to UKA for these procedures.

Geography

Geographical factors play a double role. First, proximity to national borders limits the hospitals' natural domestic catchment areas (Interviews 1, 2, 4 and 5). UKA has only a half-moon shaped hinterland and MUMC+ a narrow strip of land. The catchment area for MUMC+ has a population of around 660 000 (and shrinking – see section on "Demography" below), significantly lower than other Dutch university hospitals.

Second, the two hospitals are too close to ignore each other. Remote from other collaboration networks but with only 30 km between them, MUMC+ and UKA are obvious partners (Interview 5). Without cross-border collaboration, they would risk being in "splendid isolation" (Interview 3) or becoming "strong cross-border competitors" (Ittel, 2011; Sass and Peeters, 2008).

Demography

South Limburg faces important demographic challenges. Its population is expected to shrink by 9% between 2010 and 2025 compared with 1% and 3% in the north and central regions of the province (PRV-Limburg, 2011), and the number of inhabitants to fall to 500 000 due to lower birth rates, a rapidly ageing population, and young people leaving for the west of the Netherlands where wages and standards of living are higher (Interview 8). As a catchment area this may be too small for an academic hospital (Interviews 10 and 14). The severe health workforce shortages forecast add to the concern for hospitals in the periphery such as MUMC+ (Interviews 8, 9 and 10). The authors did not find evidence of these issues on the German side.

Competition and cooperation

In the south of the Netherlands it is not uncommon for health insurers to contract Belgian hospitals as a result of long waiting lists in the late 1990s. By late 2004 CZ and VGZ[4] had nine contracts with Belgian hospitals between them (Glinos et al., 2005). The then CEO of MUMC+ criticized the practice as "completely irresponsible" (Vollard, 2009), fearing cross-border competition and an outflowing of money. MUMC+ started developing its cross-border strategy within this climate (Interview 4), and later signed the agreement with UKA explicitly prioritizing health professional mobility. Today, Belgian hospitals continue to attract patients from South Limburg even though waiting lists are gone. CZ estimates that 3% of its local members go to Belgium (8000–9000 patients) mainly for elective care (NMa, 2012). Tongeren hospital in Belgium and Sittard hospital in the Netherlands also work together: some 200 Dutch patients annually undergo brain surgery at Tongeren, and Belgian neurosurgeons see Dutch patients with spine disorders at Sittard (Interview 13). Meanwhile, the hospital environment is changing (see also the section on "National debate" below). In 2012 the Dutch competition authority approved a merger between

---

4   CZ and VGZ are the two largest insurers in Limburg. CZ is also the largest insurer in South Limburg.

Heerlen and Sittard hospitals (see Map 7.1). The resulting "Orbis-Atrium" is expected to be among the five highest volume hospitals in the Netherlands (Interview 13). Cross-border flows to Belgium and a large, modern hospital only 25 km away increase competition considerably for MUMC+, which needs to attract complex referrals as well as basic care volumes (Interviews 6, 11 and 13; NMa, 2012). Hospitals in South Limburg are interdependent in terms of their choices of specialization, patient referrals and training of sufficient physicians in the region (PRV-Limburg, 2010): they need to maintain good relations despite fierce competition in the past (van Engelshoven, 2010; Wolf, 2004; Interview 14).

On the German side, hospitals are even more numerous and patients have considerable choice (Interviews 2 and 14). Aachen city has three hospitals, including one with a well-known vascular surgery department established prior to UKA's (Interviews 2 and 6). All German hospitals also have to respond to competition and to the threat of closing down (Interview 2).

National debate

MUMC+ and UKA are each the "youngest and smallest university hospital in their country" (Ittel, 2011; Sass and Peeters, 2008). Historically, the decision in the late 1960s to establish an eighth medical faculty in Maastricht was widely contested. Prior to the medical faculty, Maastricht had no university. At the national level some still argue that five or six university hospitals would be sufficient (Interviews 11, 13 and 14); at the regional level the choice of Maastricht over Heerlen, where a large teaching hospital providing medical training to junior specialist doctors already existed, was highly controversial (Interview 14; Wolf, 2004).

The number of hospitals in the Netherlands fell from 200 in the early 1980s to 100 in 2010 (Schäfer et al., 2010), and is expected to fall to 50 (excluding independent treatment centres) within the coming decades (Interview 13). As the newest and smallest university in a shrinking region, MUMC+ might be vulnerable (Interview 10; see also PRV-Limburg, 2010), although the hospital disputes this strongly (Interview 5). Without MUMC+, patients would have alternative options of accessing academic care in Nijmegen (143 km away) or across the border in Aachen, Liege or Leuven, even if this were detrimental to Limburg and its population (Interviews 11, 13 and 14). Maastricht University is the largest employer in the province and "plays an important role in maintaining job opportunities and promoting quality of life" (Mols, 2011). In addition, 25% of the South Limburg workforce works directly or indirectly in health care (Interview 13).

North Rhine-Westphalia held a prominent debate on whether to close academic hospital facilities some years ago, including a list of hospitals at risk (Interviews 2, 5, 14, 15 and 16).

Personal ambition

Interviewees repeatedly highlighted the role played by individuals in the collaboration (Interviews 1, 2, 3, 5, 6, 7, 10 and 14). Ambition, strong belief in cross-border collaboration and the hard work of some people at MUMC+ and UKA were instrumental in pushing it forward.

On the Dutch side, these frontrunners in their different ways made it a personal goal to make "something big" out of MUMC+, including through cross-border collaboration (Interviews 3, 5, 7 and 14). Once Maastricht obtained its university, the priority became to secure its position. The leaders of Maastricht University have tended to come from Limburg and some have been strong supporters of their native region (Interview 14; Wolf, 2004).

Obstacles and cancellation of plans

Despite the incentives to collaborate and years of preparation the hospitals officially abandoned plans for the cross-border cardiovascular centre and merger in 2012. A series of internal and external explanatory factors emerged from stakeholders' accounts; the authors complemented these findings with information from written sources where necessary.

Diverging needs and priorities

From the outset, MUMC+'s priority was to create a "centre of excellence" in cardiovascular diseases, competitive across Europe and built on a new location (Avantis). UKA wanted a hospital merger according to the "two sites, one management" model. An outright merger was impossible for MUMC+ as Dutch competition authorities view such initiatives with suspicion, while for the UKA supervisory board the idea of a new centre was a cause for concern (Interview 5). A midway solution pleased both parties to a certain extent: the cardiovascular centre became justification for the gradual merger as the joint centre would make MUMC+ and UKA interdependent, requiring one integrated decision-making structure (Interviews 5 and 10). Based on this compromise, plans went ahead for years. With hindsight, the gap in priorities was perhaps too large to bridge.

Moreover, while the two hospitals shared an interest in cardiovascular medicine, the field is losing ground to new priorities in Germany, in particular neurosciences and oncology, which receive more attention and research funding (Interview 3). Some noted that MUMC+ appeared more keenly involved in the collaboration (Interviews 3, 5 and 14).

Internal concerns

UKA apparently continued to doubt whether building a new cardiovascular centre was necessary and was uneasy about the implications of carving out departments from the parent hospitals. While the MUMC+ leadership was optimistic that net income would set in from the fourth year, UKA feared it would take longer. At MUMC+, opposition grew among medical and non-medical staff because they considered the cardiovascular departments indispensable for the hospital's academic integrity and as an income source (Interviews 3 and 5; Bos, 2009).

Questions also remained about how staff and patients would communicate and commute between the parent hospitals and the third location (Interviews 3 and 10). Some MUMC+ staff complained that collaboration distracted the leadership from "real issues" and that research (as opposed to patient care) did not receive due attention (Interviews 6 and 7). Some interviewees admitted that the frontrunners had been "walking ahead of the troops", pushing a project about which most staff on both sides were indifferent, ignorant or reluctant (Interviews 3, 5, 6, 8 and 14).

Unresolved issues and political support

A range of technical issues remained in doubt despite long negotiations between MUMC+ and UKA. These included the judicial status of the EUH as an entity of public or private law; the judicial status and exact location of the cardiovascular centre; the differences between Germany and the Netherlands in the reimbursement of patient care, medical protocols, skills of nursing staff, salary levels, staff regulations, taxation, pensions, social protection and management culture; and how to reconcile working in two administrative, funding and fiscal systems (Theisen and Heide, 2010).

Implementing the EUH and cardiovascular centre required an official agreement between the ministries of North Rhine-Westphalia and the Netherlands. The two hospitals asked their authorities to make derogations to national law, such as by replacing national planning of highly specialized services with a cross-border approach, "lightly" harmonizing medical standards, simplifying the recognition procedure of medical diplomas, granting the new centre academic status, aligning (the recognition of) nursing competences, releasing the fixed budget segment of MUMC+ to allow treatment of UKA patients, and finding creative solutions to facilitate working in two systems.[5]

Political support from the German and Dutch ministries was a "basic requirement to realize the EUH" (Ittel, 2011). Given the range and complexity of issues, numerous actors (the ministry of science and research, municipal authorities and sickness funds on the German side, and the ministries of health, education and internal affairs as well as insurers on the Dutch side) needed to endorse the project. Politicians and public authorities generally paid lip service to the cardiovascular centre and merger plans but were in practice not willing, or able, to make the necessary derogations. Nonetheless, according to the lawyers, no legal problem was irresolvable (Interviews 1, 2 and 10).

A critical decision was whether the cardiovascular centre would come under Dutch or German jurisdiction, depending on its exact location (Interview 4). With regards to language, staff would communicate in Dutch, German and English and patients would as a rule receive treatment in their mother tongue (Interviews 1 and 2; Theisen and Heide, 2010). Some suggested that language and culture could pose a problem for patients (Interviews 11 and 14; Euregio, 2012): "a German patient in the Netherlands doesn't feel comfortable and vice versa because of language issues" (Interview 3).

The business case and financial crisis

The development of the cardiovascular centre and merger plans coincided with the global financial crisis. Uncertainty about the viability of the centre's business case grew. What had seemed innovative became a high-risk, expensive project (Interviews 5, 9, 10 and 14). On the Dutch side, where banks and insurers play a major role in financing new hospital infrastructure, this made it difficult to secure the €200 million loan. Questions remained on whether it was wise to assume that patients would come from outside the usual catchment areas, including from abroad (Interviews 10 and 14).

Others argued there was no need for the centre. In the last ten years South Limburg has seen two other multimillion euro projects. Atrium Hospital (in Heerlen, 25 km east of Maastricht) underwent renovation for €150 million, downsized from the planned €300 million. Orbis Medical Centre (in Sittard, 25 km north of Maastricht) opened its doors in 2009 and cost €320 million to

---

5 Notitie n.a.v. bezoek Minister Donner. Strategisch partnerschap Maastricht UMC+ en Universitätsklinikum Aachen, aandachtspunten in de grensoverschrijdende samenwerking [Note regarding the visit of Minister (of the Interior) Donner. Strategic Partnership Maastricht UMC + and Aachen University Hospital, points on the cross-border cooperation]. Unpublished MUMC+ document, 7 July 2011.

build (see Map 7.1). Although fully operational and remarkably modern, Orbis was struggling to avoid bankruptcy, causing concern to regional insurers and national health authorities. For a region of 660 000 inhabitants, it was neither realistic nor necessary to invest in more hospital infrastructure (Interviews 11, 12, 13 and 14).

Complexity and loss of momentum

The complexity and magnitude of trying to harmonize the functioning of two hospitals in two health care systems cannot be overstated. One interviewee compared the exercise to that of merging two businesses with a €500 million turnover and some 5000 employees each, added to which are the extra complexities of medicine, cross-border health care, and the academic sector. The task was enormous, and hospitals are not able to dedicate the personnel or money to make it work. According to the lawyers, the two hospitals were "very brave" to embark on such a demanding project (Interview 10).

The complexity, internal doubts and external factors slowed things down. Talks dragged on for years (from around 2004 to 2011) causing loss of momentum (Interviews 5 and 10). With every round of elections at national, regional or local level, in Germany and the Netherlands, newly elected politicians needed convincing (Interviews 1 and 2). Collaboration fatigue appeared internally as the cardiovascular centre and merger plans absorbed time and energy in innumerable meetings producing few results (Interview 5).

New leadership and conflicting ambitions

On the German side, UKA's finances had started looking less strong compared with the mid-2000s when negotiations started. The hospital had struggled to keep budget figures positive since 2009. According to MUMC+, the priority of the newly arrived CEO was to improve the balance sheet and build relations with his staff (Interviews 5 and 6). Difficulties also seemed to arise as to how to share responsibilities and decision-making between MUMC+ and UKA within the cardiovascular centre (Interviews 3, 5 and 15).

The broader perspective

The interviews reveal an intricate situation reinforced by uncertainty and the large stakes involved. To put the findings into perspective, this section analyses who benefits from the cross-border collaboration, what role the EU played and what lessons the case study discloses.

Beneficiaries of the collaboration

In numerous border regions collaboration between health care actors serves to give patients access to local care (Bassi et al., 2001; Harant, 2003; Glinos and Baeten, 2006). The case of MUMC+ and UKA is different: their collaboration responded primarily to the need of both hospitals for market positioning and profiling. Some called this "strategic collaboration" (Interviews 1, 2 and 8).

The collaboration essentially serves two purposes. It allows MUMC+ and UKA to be less dependent on domestic catchment areas, to face competition and to reach volumes of care with greater ease. This helps "to secure [their] economic viability" (Brand et al., 2007) and strengthens their position. Second, collaborating partners can build a new identity as organizations engaged in a unique, high-profile project. The ambition to become a "European centre for state-of-the-art medicine and research" is a way to attract health professionals, researchers, students, patients and funding. Collaboration turns a peripheral disadvantage into an asset and a project of this scale brings visibility and publicity. MUMC+ and UKA became a widely known example of hospital collaboration (Busse at al., 2006; Glinos, 2011; van Ginneken and Busse, 2011). In 2007, they received a "model of good practice" award (Euregio, 2007) and later that year received a visit from the EU Commissioner for Health.

The question of who benefits is relevant because the purpose of collaboration is not necessarily (only) what partners declare or what appears. Other studies note that insurers, for example, can use contracts with foreign providers as a means to discipline domestic providers while importing capacity to address unmet demand (Baeten et al., 2006; Glinos et al., 2010; NMa, 2012). It is difficult to prove whether collaboration stimulates the economy of the wider region and brings added value to regional as well as international patients by "improving top clinical care in the Euregio Meuse-Rhine", as MUMC+ and UKA have argued (Sass and Peeters, 2008; Theisen and Heide, 2010; Scheres, 2010; Ittel, 2011). Interviewees suggested that "theoretically it should be the patient" who benefits or hoped that patients benefit (Interviews 3, 4 and 11).

Role of the EU

The EU played a complex role in the Maastricht–Aachen collaboration as a symbol and as a source of early funding, legitimacy and inspiration, but also one of disappointment. The collaboration used the EU symbolically in several ways. In 1996, the Maastricht University board decided to change the name of the former Rijksuniversiteit Limburg to "Universiteit Maastricht" to take advantage of the name of the city where the Treaty on European

Union was signed in 1992. According to one interviewee, the Maastricht name continues to be important for the "survival of the hospital" (Interview 3). Formulations such as "EUH" and "European joint centres" use Europe as a brand. That this "European" status is self-proclaimed is immaterial: Europe becomes a unique selling point to create a new identity, making what is peripheral significant. Such formulations involve stretching the label: what, for example, is "European" about two hospitals sharing a commuting nurse or a particle accelerator? Partners are less eager to create a bi-national, transnational or border region facility; creating a European centre sounds prestigious and becomes a collaboration bandwagon.

More concretely, the EU sponsored the very early steps towards collaboration. The Interreg project set up in 1991 involving UKA, MUMC+ and Liege University Hospital was among the first EU-funded projects in the health care field. The hospital collaboration also fits into the spirit of European and border region integration promoted since the 1970s by Euregio Meuse-Rhine where the university hospitals are located.

While UKA and MUMC+ did not receive EU funding for their merger and cardiovascular centre plans, they used the EU as a source of legitimacy and status, hooking their project onto EU legislation. A week after the European Commission published its proposal for a cross-border health care directive (European Commission, 2008), the two hospitals called a press conference to announce the results of the KPMG feasibility study, highlighting the fit with the "European policy context", and in particular the article on European reference networks (Sass and Peeters, 2008). The partners also emphasized the exemplary value of their collaboration, which "illustrates how European cooperation, as described in the EU Directive on patients' rights to cross-border health care, can work in practice".[6] As a pilot model for future developments, the collaboration was said to offer evidence to national and EU policy-makers (Theisen and Heide, 2010; Ittel, 2011), while pictures of the EU Commissioner and the meeting of EU health ministers were used to stress the European link. By referring to a prominent piece of EU legislation and high-profile events, the two hospitals used discursive legitimation (Vaara and Monin, 2010) to increase the status and relevance of their project, which helps to mobilize internal as well as external support.

Such a tactic can, however, entail a risk of linking projects to "fashions", which tend to come and go. The 1990s and mid-2000s when the two hospitals were preparing their ambitious plans coincided with a period of optimism and expanding European integration (the common currency launched in 2002, and preparations were under way for the 2004 accession of eight new Member

---

6 Notitie n.a.v. bezoek Minister Donner 2011 (op. cit.).

States). The context inspired cross-border collaboration and there was a general belief in things European (Interview 4). A decade later, things had drastically changed with the global financial crisis, the downturn of the European economy, and arguably shaky political support for the EU project as a whole. Several interviewees expressed disappointment that the EU had not been able actively to help the two hospitals despite giving attention and praise to the project (Interviews 1, 2, 3 and 10).

Lessons learned

Several observations with relevance for border regions emerge from the case study. One is the role of large hospitals such as MUMC+ and UKA at the regional level. As large employers, as institutions providing health care to the population, and as centres of knowledge and education, academic hospitals are "heavyweights", particularly in regions that are otherwise isolated or considered peripheral. This might explain the authors' impression that actors in South Limburg consider cross-border collaboration a bigger deal than those in North Rhine-Westphalia. Second, the respective weights of MUMC+ and UKA mean that they are too close to ignore each other. Proximity both facilitates and necessitates collaboration. At 30 km apart, their catchment areas partly coincide and it makes sense not to duplicate expensive investments.[7] Had there been no border, there might not have been two university hospitals so close together.

Yet, while the border conditions the two hospitals, it does not exempt them from national rules. Hospitals remain firmly embedded in the national health systems that fund and regulate them. The technical difficulties MUMC+ and UKA faced boil down to the tremendous – in size and number – differences between the two health systems of which they are part. For every difference, the two partners had to ask competent authorities for derogations from national rules, or to come up with inventive solutions. This made the endeavour of creating a joint centre and merging the two hospitals even more arduous: authorities are rarely keen to make exceptions, and ad hoc solutions are time consuming and unpredictable. Moreover, incentives are often national. The reasons interviewees put forward to explain the collaboration were often formed at the national level (for example, health care reforms, competition, volume criteria and history) and not necessarily specific to the border region. The misalignment of incentives between MUMC+ and UKA and the diverging views on how to collaborate were partly a result of each partner trying to tailor the collaboration according to the priorities of its health system. The hospitals' situation is not radically different from that of other hospitals working in competitive environments, and inland university hospitals

---

7   Moreover, Liege University Hospital is another 30 km away from Maastricht and 50 km from Aachen.

also collaborate with each other. This suggests that border regions might not be as exceptional as is often argued.

The question remains why the two hospitals embarked on so difficult a project. Why did they defy the technical difficulties, their diverging priorities, internal opposition and the huge costs and risks involved in a project never before tried anywhere else? Is it, for example, realistic to expect public authorities to make derogations to national laws? One hypothesis is that of hubris developed by Roll (1986) to explain why decision-makers in corporate takeovers overestimate gains and convince themselves that their valuation is correct. In the UKA–MUMC+ setting elements suggest that overconfidence (hubris) among the collaboration frontrunners contributed to a crisis resulting in the breakdown of plans (nemesis). In their effort to sell the project, they overlooked the obstacles. That the collaboration did not respond to a clear need of the local population might have reinforced the mechanism of overconfidence and advocating collaboration.

Whether or not this is the case, it seems clear that ambitious plans were the personal project of a small group of individuals who saw the benefits collaboration could bring in terms of prestige and preparedness for the future at both the institutional and personal levels. They pushed the collaboration forward and sought to convince others of its merits. Without them, collaboration might never have taken off or developed.

A last important observation is that collaboration between institutions can take place at several levels simultaneously. Daily cross-border working between the two hospitals' medical teams and departments continues seemingly undisturbed by the cancellation of grander plans. Two months after the cancellation, UKA renewed the contract of the commuting vascular professor. This indicates that pragmatic collaboration serving an objective purpose and with tangible results for those involved can outlive high-flying ambitions.

Conclusion

This is a story of two university hospitals too close to ignore each other. A complex mix of parameters led UKA and MUMC+ to collaborate. Unfavourable geography, small and shrinking catchment areas, minimum volume requirements set at national levels, increasingly demanding environments in which university hospitals must specialize and invest to compete nationally and Europe-wide, as well as a handful of dynamic individuals, formed the set of challenges and opportunities that reinforced each other to create a setting where collaborating seemed an obvious course. In contrast to other examples of cross-border collaboration, that between UKA and MUMC+ was not driven by the need of local patients to access care, but rather by the strategic considerations of the two partners seeking to position themselves in a competitive setting and to create a new profile as a joint EUH.

The two hospitals faced internal as well as external obstacles on their way to collaboration. Late 2011 saw the cancellation of plans for the construction of a new cross-border facility and a hospital merger involving numerous practical, legal and financial issues to be resolved. The complexity of the endeavour, high costs, high risks, unclear need and far-reaching consequences for UKA and MUMC+ meant the abandonment of the radical approach to collaboration. Concrete, day-to-day collaboration, however, seems to persist between medical teams and departments, suggesting that where there is a real need, collaboration continues.

References

azM (2012). *Nieuwbouw op Avantis van de baan [New building at Avantis cancelled]* [press release]. Maastricht, academisch ziekenhuis Maastricht (www.azm.nl/hetazm/nieuws/224927, accessed 20 December 2012).

Baeten R, McKee M, Rosenmöller M (2006). Conclusions. In: Rosenmöller M, McKee M, Baeten R, eds. *Patient mobility in the European Union: learning from experience.* Copenhagen, WHO Regional Office for Europe: 179–87 (www.euro.who.int/__data/assets/pdf_file/0005/98420/Patient_Mobility.pdf, accessed 17 June 2013).

Bassi D, Deuert O, Garel P, Ortiz A (2001). *An assessment of cross-border cooperation between hospitals: France – Belgium - Luxembourg – Germany – Italy – Spain – Great Britain – Switzerland.* Paris, Mission opérationelle transfrontalière (www.espaces-transfrontaliers.org/document/santeanglais.pdf, accessed 20 December 2012).

Bos W (2009). Groeiende onrust over Avantis-plan: "Cardiologie eruit, dat kan niet" [Growing unease with Avantis plan: "Cardiology leaving, that won't do"]. *Observant*, 22 October (www.observantonline.nl/Archief/ArtikelenOud/tabid/69/agentType/View/PropertyID/798/Default.aspx, accessed 20 December 2012).

Bos W (2012). Hart- en vaatziektencentrum op Avantis aan zijden draad [Heart and vascular centre at Avantis hanging by a thread]. *Observant*, 5 January (www.observantonline.nl/Archief/ArtikelenOud/tabid/69/agentType/View/PropertyID/3998/Default.aspx, accessed 20 December 2012).

Brand H, Hollederer A, Ward G, Wolf U (2007). *Evaluation of border regions in the European Union (EUREGIO), Final Report.* Brussels, European Commission (http://ec.europa.eu/health/ph_projects/2003/action1/docs/2003_1_23_frep_en.pdf, accessed 20 December 2012).

Brand H, Hollederer A, Wolf U, Brand A (2008). Cross-border health activities in the Euregios: good practice for better health. *Health Policy,* 86(2–3): 245–54.

Busse R, Woerz M, Foubister T, Mossialos E, Berman P (2006). *Mapping health services access: national and cross-border issues (HealthACCESS). Final report.* Brussels, European Health Management Association (http://ec.europa.eu/health/ph_projects/2003/action1/docs/2003_1_22_frep_en.pdf, accessed 20 December 2012).

Doering N, Legido-Quigley H, Glinos IA, McKee M, Maarse H (2013). A success-story in cross-border telemedicine in Europe: the use of intra-operative teleneuromonitoring during aorta surgery. *Health Policy and Technology,* 2(1): 4–9.

empirica GmbH (2004). *Case study: cross-border cooperation in health care provision in Euregio Meuse-Rhine.* Bonn, e-business Watch/European Commission, DG Enterprise & Industry (http://ec.europa.eu/enterprise/archives/e-business-watch/studies/case_studies/documents/Case%20Studies%202004/CS_SR10_Health_2-Euregio.pdf, accessed 20 December 2012).

Euregio (2007). Final Conference of the "EUREGIO" Project on 6 March 2007 in Düsseldorf: "Cross-Border Activities – Good Practice for Better Health" [web site]. Düsseldorf, Landesinstitut für Gesundheit und Arbeit NRW (www.euregio.nrw.de/downloads_conference07.html, accessed 20 December 2012).

Euregio (2012). *Guideline for the use of health technology assessment in cross border settings: a deliverable for the project – solutions for improving health care cooperation in border regions (Euregio ii Work Package 5).* Maastricht, Maastricht University (www.euregio2-conference.eu/info/General/WP5.pdf, accessed 28 June 2013).

European Commission (2008). *Proposal for a Directive of the European Parliament and of the Council on the application of patients' rights in cross-border health care. COM (2008) 414 final.* Brussels, European Commission (http://ec.europa.eu/health/ph_overview/co_operation/healthcare/docs/COM_en.pdf, accessed 28 June 2013).

Glinos IA (2011). Cross-border collaboration. In: Wismar M, Palm W, Figueras J, Ernst K and Van Ginneken E, eds. *Cross-border health care in the European Union: mapping and analysing practices and policies.* Copenhagen, WHO Regional Office for Europe on behalf of the European Observatory on Health Systems and Policies (Observatory Studies Series, No. 22: 217–54; www.euro.who.int/__data/assets/pdf_file/0004/135994/e94875.pdf, accessed 20 December 2012).

Glinos IA, Baeten R (2006). *A literature review of cross-border patient mobility in the European Union.* Brussels, Observatoire social européen (www.ose.be/files/publication/health/WP12_lit_review_final.pdf, accessed 20 December 2012).

Glinos IA, Boffin N, Baeten R (2005). *Contracting cross-border care in Belgian hospitals: an analysis of Belgian, Dutch and English stakeholder perspectives.* Brussels, Obscrvatoire social européen (www.ose.be/files/publication/2005/baeten_glinos_2005_BelgianCaseStudy.pdf, accessed 20 December 2012).

Glinos IA, Baeten R, Maarse H (2010). Purchasing health services abroad: practices of cross-border contracting and patient mobility in six European countries. *Health Policy*, 95(2–3): 103–12.

Harant P (2003). Hospital cooperation in border regions in Europe. In: *Free movement and cross-border cooperation in Europe: the role of hospitals and practical experiences in hospitals, proceedings of the HOPE Conference and Workshop, Luxembourg, June 2003.* Luxembourg, Entente des hôpitaux luxembourgeois: 34–7.

Hermans H, den Exter A (1999). Cross-border alliances in health care: international co-operation between health insurers and providers in the Euregio Meuse-Rhine. *Croatian Medical Journal*, 40(2): 266–72.

Ittel T (2011). University Hospital Aachen – how to manage a growing European perspective [presentation]. *Hospital Build Europe 2011 Exhibition and Congress, Conference 3: Leaders in healthcare, Nuremberg, 4–5 April.*

Maastricht UMC+ (2010). *Heel de mens – Een eerste kennismaking met Maastricht UMC+ [Heal the human – a first encounter with Maastricht UMC+]* [corporate brochure]. Maastricht, MUMC+ (www.heritage.azm.nl/afbeeldingen/download/heeldemensazm/flash.html#/1/, accessed 27 June 2013).

Maastricht University (2009). Important dates [web site]. Maastricht, Maastricht University (www.maastrichtuniversity.nl/web/Main/AboutUM/ History/ImportantDates.htm, accessed 20 December 2012).

Mols G (2011). We are an international teaching and research university, *Maastricht University Magazine*, 03 October. Maastricht, Maastricht University: 3 (http://issuu.com/maastrichtuniversity/docs/um_magazine_ october_2011, accessed 27 June 2013).

NMa (2012). *Besluit van de Raad van Bestuur van de Nederlandse Mededingingsautoriteit in Artikel 41 van de Mededinginswet. Nummer 7236/659. Betreft zaak: 7236/ Orbis-Atrium. [Decision of the Executive Board of the Dutch Competition Authority under Art. 41 of the Competition Law. Number 7236/659. Concerning case: 7236/ Orbis-Atrium]* The Hague, Nederlandse Mededingingsautoriteit (www.acm.nl/nl/download/ publicatie/?id=10909, accessed 26 June 2013).

Palm W, Glinos IA, Garel P, Busse R, Rechel B, Figueras J, eds. (2013). *Building European reference networks: exploring concepts and national practices in the European Union.* Copenhagen, WHO Regional Office for Europe on behalf of the European Observatory on Health Systems and Policies (Observatory Studies Series, No. 28; www.euro.who.int/__data/assets/ pdf_file/0004/184738/e96805-final.pdf, accessed 20 December 2012).

PRV-Limburg (2010). *Een gezamenlijke toekomst voor ziekenhuiszorg in Limburg [A shared future for hospital care in Limburg].* Maastricht, Provinciale Raad voor de Volksgezondheid Limburg (www.prv-limburg.nl/sites/ prv-limburg.nl/files/adviezen/Een%20gezamenlijke%20toekomst%20 voor%20ziekenhuiszorg%20in%20Limburg%2001-06-2010.pdf, accessed 27 June 2013).

PRV-Limburg (2011). *Limburg op leeftijd. Zorg en ondersteuning in tijden van bevolkingskrimp. Advies over de toekomst van zorg en voorzieningen voor ouderen [Limburg on age. Care and support in times of population decline. Opinion on the future of health care and services for the elderly].* Maastricht, Provinciale Raad voor de Volksgezondheid Limburg (www.prv-limburg.nl/ sites/prv-limburg.nl/files/adviezen/Advies%20Toekomst%20van%20de%20 Zorg%20in%20Limburg%20december%202011.pdf, accessed 27 June 2013).

Roll R (1986). The hubris hypothesis of corporate takeovers. *Journal of Business*, 59(2, pt 1): 197–216.

Sass H and Peeters G (2008). *Ergebnisse der Machbarkeitsstudie uber die Zusammenarbeit zwischen der Universitätsklinik Maastricht und dem Universitätsklinikum Aachen [Results of the feasibility study on cooperation between University Hospital Maastricht and University Hospital Aachen]* [Presentation given at press conference, 8 July]. Aachen, Universitätsklinikum Aachen (www.uk-aachen.de/go/show?ID=6389229&DV=0&COMP= download&NAVID=6389151&NAVDV=0, accessed 27 June 2013).

Schäfer W, Kroneman M, Boerma W, van den Berg M, Westert G, Devillé W, van Ginneken E (2010). The Netherlands: health system review. *Health Systems in Transition*, 12(1): 1–229 Copenhagen, WHO Regional Office for Europe (www.euro.who.int/__data/assets/pdf_file/0008/85391/E93667.pdf, accessed 27 June 2013).

Scheres J (2010). The failed (dclayed) patients' directive, the 883/2004 Regulation and their implications on cross border health care in border regions. *Euregio ii project partners meeting, Cologne, 19–20 May 2010* (www.maastrichtuniversity.nl/web/file?uuid=743ee670-90b5-41bb-842d-2233d9d36a95&owner=c3132aeb-833f-41b1-8c26-71815914b200, accessed 20 December 2012).

Summum actueel (2010). Prof. Dr Mottaghy benoemd tot nieuw afdelingshoofd nucleaire geneeskunde [Professor Mottaghy named new head of nuclear medicine department]. *Summum actueel* [internal hospital newsletter], 5(3): 3, June.

Theisen S, Heide A (2010). *Presentation: Kooperation Universitaetsklinikum Aachen & Maastricht UMC+ [Cooperation between University Hospital Aachen and Maastricht UMC+]*, 16 June 2010.

UKA (2007). *Machbarkeitsstudie für ein Europäisches Universitätsklinikum [Feasibility study for a European University Hospital]*, Aachen, UKA Office of Corporate Communications (www.uk-aachen.de/go/changelanguage?ID= 5191106&DV=3&COMP=page&NAVID=5191106&NAVDV=3, accessed 26 June 2013).

Vaara E and Monin P (2010). A recursive perspective on discursive legitimation and organizational action in mergers and acquisitions. *Organization Science*, 21(1): 3–22.

van Engelshoven, JMA (2010). Taakverdeling en concentratie in ziekenhuiszorg noodzaak [The need for task distribution and concentration hospital care]. In: PRV-Limburg. *Een gezamenlijke toekomst voor ziekenhuiszorg in Limburg [A shared future for hospital care in Limburg]*. Maastricht, Provinciale Raad voor de Volksgezondheid Limburg: 115–24.

van Ginneken E and Busse R (2011). Cross-border health care data. In: Wismar M, Palm W, Figueras J, Ernst K and Van Ginneken E, eds. *Cross-border health care in the European Union: mapping and analysing practices and policies*. Copenhagen, WHO Regional Office for Europe (Observatory Studies Series, No. 22: 289–340; www.euro.who.int/__data/assets/ pdf_file/0004/135994/e94875.pdf, accessed 20 December 2012).

Vollard H (2009). Cross-border patient mobility in the European Union and the Netherlands. In: *Political territoriality in the European Union: the changing boundaries of security and health care* [PhD thesis]. Leiden University: 347–408.

Wolf, R. (2004). *Mijn Ziekenhuis – 100 jaar ziekenhuiszorg in Parkstad Limburg [My hospital – 100 years of hospital care in Parkstad Limburg]*. Heerlen, Bureau PR Atrium MC.

Annex 7.1 Interviews conducted

Number	Date	Interviewee	Institution
Actors with a central role in the collaboration			
Interview 1	23 February 2012 (joint interview)	Management/ executive level	MUMC+
Interview 2		Management/ executive level	UKA
Interview 3	8 March 2012	Head of medical departments	MUMC+ and UKA
Interview 4	12 March 2012	Management/ executive level	MUMC+
Interview 5	25 April 2012	Management/ executive level	MUMC+
Interview 6	26 September 2012	Management/ executive level	MUMC+
Staff with no active role in the collaboration			
Interview 7	8 February 2012	Researcher	Maastricht University
Interview 8	28 March 2012	Representative from nursing staff association	MUMC+
Interview 9	3 April 2012	Human resources adviser	MUMC+
External observers			
Interview 10	15 February 2012	Legal advisers (two)	VMW law firm, the Netherlands
Insurers			
Interview 11	25 April 2012	Officer, contracting dept.	Insurance company, the Netherlands
Interview 12	26 September 2012	Officer, contracting dept.	Insurance company, the Netherlands
Potential competitors			
Interview 13	7 March 2012	Director	Hospital, South Limburg, the Netherlands
Interview 14	9 March 2012	Former director	Hospital, South Limburg, the Netherlands
Interview 15	22 March 2012	Commercial director	University hospital, North Rhine-Westphalia, Germany
Interview 16	30 March 2012	Commercial director	University hospital, North Rhine-Westphalia, Germany

Annex 7.2 Stakeholders unavailable for interview

Date of requests	Position	Institution
March 2012	Member of medical staff association	MUMC+
March–May 2012	Management/executive level	UKA
March 2012	Medical director and commercial director	University hospital, North Rhine-Westphalia, Germany
April–May 2012	Director	Hospital, Aachen, North Rhine-Westphalia, Germany
April–May 2012	Director	Hospital, Aachen, North Rhine-Westphalia, Germany
April–May 2012	Member of ministerial council	Ministry of Innovation, Science and Research, North Rhine-Westphalia, Germany

Chapter 8

Working across the Danube: Călăraşi and Silistra hospitals sharing doctors (Romania–Bulgaria)

Adriana Galan, Victor Olsavszky and Cristian Vlădescu

Introduction

In March 2011 the WHO Regional Office for Europe organized a Technical Meeting on Health Workforce Retention in countries of the South-eastern Europe Health Network, held in Bucharest. The Romanian meeting participants were surprised to learn from their Bulgarian counterparts that physicians living in Bulgaria crossed the Danube by ferry to work night shifts in Romania (WHO, 2011). This chapter investigates the new phenomenon for the Romanian health care system: the inflow of foreign doctors in the context of cross-border mobility and their active recruitment by a large district hospital.

Cross-border mobility in the district of Călăraşi, a south-eastern region of Romania bordering Bulgaria, mainly involves the movement of health care professionals in one direction from Bulgaria to Romania. This responds to the very acute problem of a shortage of physicians in Romanian hospitals, which stems from a combination of factors including emigration flows since the country's accession to the European Union (EU), as well as salary cuts and recruitment freezes in the public health care sector as part of measures to counteract the economic crisis.

The collaboration instigated by Călăraşi District Emergency Hospital (DEH) involves contractual agreements with individual Bulgarian physicians rather than other hospitals or health authorities. The Romanian hospital has a severe staffing shortage in some areas and actively seeks to recruit specialist doctors – in particular anaesthetists – from Bulgaria and the Republic of Moldova. On the other side of the Danube, some 2 km away, Silistra Hospital in Bulgaria has a surplus of anaesthetists. Five Bulgarian physicians work at both locations, travelling across the river around five times per month to complete a 24-hour shift at Călăraşi DEH, having reduced their working hours at Silistra Hospital.

The arrangement brings clear benefits for the Romanian hospital. For the Bulgarian provider the cross-border commuting alleviates internal pressures, reduces salary expenses and offers the advantage that its specialists do not leave the national health system. Increased earnings are an incentive for the commuting doctors: despite a 25% salary cut in the Romanian public health care sector since 2010 (recovered only in December 2012), wages remain attractive compared with those in Bulgaria. This chapter offers further insight into the impact of the cross-border collaboration on the health systems.

Methodology

To evaluate the collaboration the authors combined desk research and interviews with key informants. They drew up a list of experts and stakeholders during the preparatory research stage, including actors with important roles in the management of human resources for health at the local level: managers of Călăraşi DEH and the district public health directorate (DPHD) and representatives of the physicians from Bulgaria. The initial list also included members of the Călăraşi District Health Insurance Fund and Călăraşi District College of Physicians. With help from the DPHD, the authors scheduled three interviews at Călăraşi DEH (with the hospital's general manager, a Bulgarian doctor and the head of the intensive care unit) and two interviews with the executive director and the head of the Health Status Evaluation and Health Promotion Department of Călăraşi DPHD, a Bulgarian doctor and the head of the intensive care unit (see Annex 8.1 for interview details). Nobody declined an interview request, and the interviewees provided all the necessary information, so further interviews with representatives of the health insurance fund and College of Physicians were not required.

The Călăraşi DEH general manager, Dr Victor Verinceanu, was of particular assistance in analysing the collaboration (Interview 3). He initiated the headhunting process to overcome the chronic shortage of staff in some specialties in his organization, having dedicated his professional life to health care delivery and management in Călăraşi.

The authors developed a semi-structured interview questionnaire based on three major research questions:

- How does the hospital collaboration work?
- Why does it exist?
- What is the role of the EU in the collaboration?

They performed face-to-face interviews, during which they took written notes. During the field visit to Călăraşi DEH they also collected quantitative data on the number and distribution of hospital doctors by specialty and department, as well as financial details on the average income of the Bulgarian doctors.

Context and evolution of the Călăraşi DEH collaboration

The region and its health care system

Romania is located at the crossroads of central and south-eastern Europe on the Lower Danube, bordering the Black Sea. It shares borders with Hungary and Serbia to the west, Ukraine and the Republic of Moldova to the north-east and east, and Bulgaria to the south. At 238 400 km² Romania is the ninth largest country by area in the EU, and has the seventh largest population, at 21.4 million according to the Ministry of Health (2011), although according to preliminary data from the 2011 census, the population of Romania is only 20.1 million people.

The border between Romania and Bulgaria – first established in 1878 and changing its shape and length over time, but remaining fixed since the Craiova Treaty of 1940[1] – measures 631.3 km. Most of it (470 km) follows the Danube watercourse (Map 8.1). The cities of Călăraşi in Romania and Silistra in Bulgaria lie at the end point of the river border, some 2 km apart. A ferry crosses the river every 30–45 minutes to link the two cities; the crossing takes around 20 minutes.

Map 8.1. *The Danube river border between Romania and Bulgaria (Călăraşi and Silistra circled)*

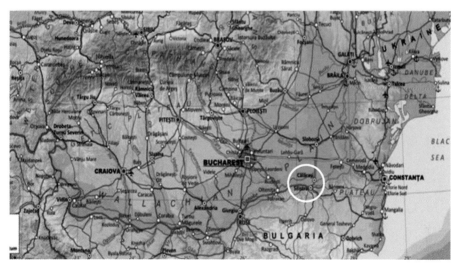

Source: Authors' own compilation

---

1 Ratification of the Treaty between Romania and Bulgaria signed at Craiova (No. 212/1940).

Călăraşi city is the capital of the district of Călăraşi, an area of about 5088 km² whose southern and eastern sides border the valley of the Danube. According to official estimates, in 2009 the district had a population of 312 879 inhabitants, 38.5% living in urban and 61.5% in rural areas (Călăraşi District Council, 2012). Călăraşi city has about 73 500 inhabitants. The local terrain is flat and the district's main economic activity is agriculture. Since industrial investment began only in recent years, the population of the district of Călăraşi has historically searched for higher-paid jobs, especially in Italy and Spain shortly after 2007 (the year Romania joined the EU). It seems now, however, that the district's population has stabilized.

The Romanian health system has two main levels: national/central and district. The national level is responsible for attaining general health objectives and ensuring the fundamental principles of the government health policy. The district level is responsible for ensuring service provision according to the rules set centrally, most notably by the Ministry of Health and the national health insurance fund. A total of 42 DPHDs operate as decentralized units of the Ministry of Health. Similarly, the national health insurance fund has 42 district health insurance fund branches. DPHDs control less than a third of the available public funds; the remainder is under the management of the district health insurance funds. Hospitals receive prospective budgets consisting of a mixture of payment methods, but mainly based on a diagnosis-related group (DRG) mechanism. From the hospital budget, the health personnel are paid salaries in all public hospitals. Most hospitals are (still) under public ownership, with very few initiatives of private practice (Vlădescu et al., 2008).

Călăraşi DEH: vacancies and shortages

In 2009 the district of Călăraşi offered inpatient care for its population through six hospitals (including one rural hospital) and two medicosocial care units (National Institute of Statistics, 2010). Like all other districts in Romania, it has a DEH in its capital city, providing health care services for the entire regional population.

The Ministry of Health decided to close 67 local hospitals that it considered inefficient across the country in April 2011. The list included the urban hospital in Budeşti (in the district of Călăraşi); for about 40 000 inhabitants their closest hospital thus became Călăraşi DEH, about 100 km from Budeşti. Nevertheless, Călăraşi District Council proposed that the Ministry of Health re-open the hospital in Budeşti as an external department of Călăraşi DEH. The proposal awaits Ministry of Health approval (Stroe, 2011).

Data obtained from Călăraşi DEH show that the hospital has 60 practising physicians and 28 junior doctors involved in specialty training programmes. Table 8.1 shows the distribution of medical specialties among these. At first glance, this highlights that some important specialties are missing, including endocrinology, haematology, pneumology, radiotherapy, different types of surgical specialty and urology, among others. The data do not reveal various other important shortages, however. They also shed no light on the new phenomenon for the Romanian health care system of the inflow of foreign physicians, mostly from neighbouring countries.

The interviewees from Călăraşi offered deeper insight into these figures. For example, although the data declare six anaesthesiology specialists, in fact the hospital has only two Romanian anaesthetists, one of whom is unwilling to work night shifts. The rest are commuting Bulgarian doctors working a 24-hour shift around five times a month. Only one practising cardiologist works at Călăraşi DEH at present but the doctor is approaching retirement, so the hospital will have no fully trained cardiology specialist; the previous cardiologist left in May 2012. The hospital's sole infectious diseases specialist is on a six-month secondment to a hospital in Bucharest, and is very likely to continue to work in Bucharest after that contract finishes. Călăraşi DEH has lacked a specialist in endocrinology for more than 10 years, during which time it has redirected all patients requiring care in this field to Bucharest, which is 130 km away. It also has no diabetes specialist: four internal medicine practitioners in ambulatory care cover this field at present, but the diabetes service is unaccredited because of the lack of a specialist. The hospital has only one oncology specialist, who is also unwilling to work night shifts.

Călăraşi DEH currently has a very tense working environment because, thanks to these personnel shortages, all doctors are obliged to work night shifts (although exemptions can be made; for example, during pregnancy or as a result of a health condition) as well as their contracted daytime hours. Moreover, interviewees from the DPHD provided a shocking estimate: the hospital lost around 200 health care personnel, especially physicians and nurses, within a period of only 18 months during 2010–2011 (Interviews 1 and 2).

In addition to this difficult situation, the hospital's general manager disclosed another sensitive issue: the maternity department is also unaccredited because it has no official neonatologist (Interview 3). A Bulgarian doctor is providing care in this specialty, but has no clear contract because her basic specialty is paediatrics, with a competence in neonatology, so she needs to attend specialist training in Romania before obtaining accreditation. In fact, many Romanian women living in the villages on the southern bank of the Danube (Călăraşi being just north of the river) deliver in Silistra because geographical access is easier and the quality of care is good. Silistra city lies on the southern side of the river where the border diverges from the Danube's course, and is closer to these Romanian villages than Călăraşi city. These women pay out of pocket for the care received at Silistra Hospital and receive reimbursement from the Călăraşi health insurance fund. Bulgarian doctors working at both hospitals have helped to facilitate this patient mobility.

Table 8.1. *Distribution of medical specialties in Călăraşi DEH, December 2011*

Medical specialty	Physicians	Specialty trainees	Total	Beds
Anaesthesiology and intensive care	6	4	10	25
Cardiology	1	2	3	40
Cardiovascular surgery			0	
Dermatology	3	0	3	10
Emergency care	2	4	6	
Endocrinology			0	
Epidemiology	1	1	2	
Forensic medicine	2	0	2	
Gastroenterology	1	0	1	
General surgery	6	1	7	75
Geriatrics	1	1	2	25
Haematology			0	
Infectious diseases	1	1	2	25
Internal medicine	3	1	4	70+2a
Laboratory	0	2	2	
Neonatology	1	2	3	30
Nephrology	1	0	1	5
Neurology	2	1	3	32
Neurosurgery			0	
Obstetrics/gynaecology	6	0	6	47
Occupational health	0	1	1	
Oncology	1	1	2	30
Ophthalmology	2	0	2	5
Oral surgery			0	
Orthopaedics	3	0	3	30
Otorhinolaryngology	2	0	2	10
Paediatric psychiatry	0	1	1	
Paediatric surgery	2	0	2	
Paediatrics	4	0	4	65

Medical specialty	Physicians	Specialty trainees	Total	Beds
Pathological anatomy	1	1	2	
Plastic surgery	2	1	3	10
Pneumology			0	
Psychiatry	2	0	2	25
Public health			0	
Radiology and imagistics	3	1	4	
Radiotherapy			0	
Rehabilitation, balneology	1	1	2	10
Rheumatology			0	
Thoracic surgery			0	
Urology			0	
Total	**60**	**28**	**88**	**571**

Source: Călărași DEH data, at authors' request.
a The two additional beds are for peritoneal dialysis.

The nursing situation, on the other hand, is very different: the three private nursing schools in Călărași district produce a high number of qualified staff, and there is thus great mobility of nurses going abroad to work for pre-determined periods of time, after which they return to Romania. These nurses retain their positions in the hospital while they are abroad, which means that the hospital does not have to lose the vacant posts, according to existing regulations.

Recruiting foreign physicians

The attempt to attract Bulgarian doctors to work at Călărași DEH began in early 2008, initiated by the Romanian side, in order to overcome the severe staff shortages in important medical specialties. Dr Verinceanu, the hospital's manager, met a Bulgarian interpreter living in Călărași, whose brother worked at Silistra Hospital as an anaesthetist. The Romanian bemoaned his hospital's shortage of anaesthetists and the Bulgarian complained of the very low salaries in the health care system in Bulgaria: this led Dr Verinceanu to initiate the recruitment drive and invite the interpreter's brother to be the first Bulgarian anaesthetist to work night shifts in Romania. Thereafter, the headhunting process continued among Bulgarian doctors from Silistra with the help of this initial recruit. He advertised possible jobs in Romania, at a higher pay rate than those in Bulgaria, and introduced more Bulgarian doctors who began work in the Romanian hospital.

By December 2011 five Bulgarian doctors (four anaesthetists and one specialist in radiology and imagistics) worked under contract at Călăraşi DEH. The hospital was also in negotiations with a Bulgarian neonatologist (who began work at the Romanian hospital in May 2012). Consequently, the hospital is currently able to ensure high-quality continuity of care for the surgery and intensive care departments.

The Bulgarian doctors' contracts stipulate the number of shifts they have to work monthly, the taxes they have to pay to the state of Romania and the Romanian work legislation they must obey. On average they work five to six 24-hour shifts each month (08:00 to 08:00), with an average net monthly income of about 1600 Romanian Leu (about €375).

The interviews also revealed that doctors from the Republic of Moldova provide cover for some important specialties at the Romanian hospital (Interview 3). Five Moldovan doctors work at Călăraşi DEH covering neurology, orthopaedics, gastroenterology, nephrology and dermatology. Theirs is a different situation, however: they graduated from Romania's Medical University and hold Romanian as well as Moldovan citizenship. Unlike their Bulgarian colleagues, the Moldovan doctors work full time at the hospital and do not need diploma recognition for accreditation.

Practical problems and solutions of cross-border recruiting

At present, Călăraşi DPHD has no power to influence policy on human resources for health at the district hospital level. Nevertheless, based on the close long-term link between the DEH and the DPHD, the latter facilitates local relationships between the hospital management and other national or local stakeholders.

The process of hiring Bulgarian physicians was not a simple one in the beginning. The first problems encountered were in obtaining diploma recognition and organizing transport from Silistra to Călăraşi. The transport issue was easier and faster to solve: the DPHD facilitated a partnership between the hospital and the border police, who agreed to offer their transport boat for the Bulgarian doctors' river crossings. A hospital car then takes the doctors from the river pier to Călăraşi DEH. When the border police boat is not available, the hospital has agreed to cover the cost of the ferry that links Călăraşi and Silistra. In general, the journey takes about 45 minutes.

The DPHD represents the interface between the Ministry of Health and Călăraşi DEH in the process of diploma recognition or certification of competence for Bulgarian doctors. The process was unclear at the beginning and has proved very time consuming. The hospital human resources department sends the doctor's documentation to Călăraşi DPHD, which forwards it to the Ministry of Health, which is in charge of granting official recognition. Once the Ministry of Health has issued a recognition certificate, the College of Physicians also has to check all the documentation, so the DPHD sends the diploma and all the competence, specialty and recognition certificates to Călăraşi District College of Physicians to obtain accreditation and the Bulgarian doctor's right to practise in Romania. Registration with the College is obligatory for all doctors in Romania, and only after the College has issued a licence to practise can a Bulgarian doctor sign a contract with Călăraşi DEH.

Thanks to its excellent relationship with the local branch of the College of Physicians, the hospital often manages to obtain these licences quickly, but the Ministry of Health still has to re-certify them each year. Călăraşi DPHD plays an important role in this process of certification and accreditation by putting pressure on the accrediting institutions to speed up the process. The normal time lag between application and accreditation may be up to a year,[2] but the DPHD's efforts can cut it to just a few months, during which time the foreign doctors cannot officially work in Romania.

Călăraşi DEH faced another problem when Bulgarian doctors started work: the language barrier (Interview 3). Romanian is a Latin language, while Bulgarian is Slavic. To overcome this new problem, the hospital employed an interpreter to work the same shifts as the Bulgarian physicians, although one Bulgarian doctor speaks very good Romanian and has no need of translation services.

Stakeholder perspectives

All the stakeholders interviewed had a positive perception of the inflow of foreign physicians into the Romanian health care system. The collaboration appeared to offer a win–win solution because the visiting doctors also solved their economic problems without having to leave their homes and families in Bulgaria.

District health authorities

Călăraşi DPHD, like all other DPHDs in Romania, plays an important role in health workforce planning, advising the Ministry of Health annually on the number of doctors and nurses needed at district level, by specialty. The situation is extremely difficult at present because since 2009 Emergency Ordinance

---

2   After Romania's accession to the EU in 2007 the Romanian Ministry of Health was overwhelmed by requests for diploma recognition from doctors already living in EU countries or willing to move to those countries: dealing with all of them became a lengthy process.

34/2009[3] – a measure to counteract the economic crisis – has prevented the filling of vacant posts in all public institutions, including health care units. It is therefore very difficult to employ new staff in the health care system. Even if the hospital succeeds in recruiting specialty trainees (resident doctors), they tend to leave the hospital soon after, or even during, the training period in order to work abroad. The DPHD's executive director called Călăraşi DEH a "springboard to work abroad" for young Romanian doctors (Interview 1), as this is such a common phenomenon. Călăraşi district also suffers in this regard from its proximity to Bucharest, which attracts an important number of personnel in various fields.

Călăraşi Health Insurance Fund, which provides the majority of DEH's funding, has also supported the hospital fully in its endeavours to employ foreign doctors to cover the staff deficit. The support of both these major institutions shows that official health care actors at the district level acknowledge the acute need to find solutions to Călăraşi DEH's health workforce problems.

Călăraşi DEH and the population it serves

The general manager described in detail the difficult situation created by the shortage of health care personnel for Călăraşi's main hospital (Interview 3). The economic crisis and the measures taken to reduce its effects by the Romanian government since 2009 have deeply affected the health care system. In 2010 the government implemented Law 118/2010,[4] which cut salaries across the whole public sector by 25%, affecting hospital personnel and many others nationwide. This was an additional reason for dissatisfaction among physicians and nurses already unhappy with the low level of salaries in the health service. The economic crisis, high level of uncertainty and lack of adequate management and planning mechanisms for human resources for health created a very demotivated health workforce; this led to high outflows of Romanian health professionals after EU accession in January 2007 (Galan et al., 2011). The situation is even worse in Călăraşi district, which is not a very economically attractive area. Staff shortages at Călăraşi DEH have also led to excessive workloads for remaining doctors, including the widespread use of night shifts to cope with the burden.

Given this difficult situation, foreign recruitment became inevitable. Thanks to the inflow of specialist doctors from Bulgaria and the Republic of Moldova, Călăraşi DEH is able at present to ensure a high quality of continuity of care for

---

3 Emergency Ordinance 34/2009 to regulate some fiscal measures (No. 249/14.04.2009).

4 Law 118/2010 regarding some necessary measures to better balance the budget (No. 878/28.12.2010).

the surgery and intensive care departments, as well as other medical disciplines. This has clear advantages in terms of access to specialized care for local patients who would otherwise have to travel 130 km to Bucharest.

Foreign physicians

Despite the cuts in salary levels, working in Romania is still financially attractive for Bulgarian doctors (Box 8.1). According to the Bulgarian Doctors' Union, the monthly salary of an anaesthetist in Bulgaria is about 700–800 Bulgarian Lev (about €350–400), representing the same amount they can earn in Romania working only around five 24-hour shifts per month (Novinite, 2011). As salary levels are also generally lower in the Republic of Moldova than Romania, similar incentives encourage Moldovan doctors to work in the neighbouring country, although different diploma and specialty recognition regulations apply for them after 2007.

Local physicians

Romanian doctors at Călăraşi DEH were initially reluctant to accept the first Bulgarian doctor working at their hospital. The relationship improved slowly over time, but only became fully trusting when a Bulgarian surgeon working as an anaesthetist in Romania solved a very difficult case. Bulgarian doctors have now built a real team with their peers and the nurses in Romania. At the end of their shifts doctors from both countries meet to discuss patient safety issues that have arisen. There is a very dynamic exchange of practice standards and knowledge; for instance, Bulgarian doctors introduced some of their national emergency care standards at the Călăraşi DEH.

Silistra Hospital

In order to prevent a potential conflict with the College of Physicians from Bulgaria related to the number of working hours per month, the Bulgarian doctors preferred to reduce their working hours at Silistra Hospital. Since the Bulgarian hospital does not lack anaesthetists, the management has accepted its doctors' mobility. In fact, only one Bulgarian doctor is missing from Silistra Hospital per day, thus not jeopardizing continuity of care. By late 2011, however, there was still no formal communication between the two hospitals across the river border.

Box 8.1. *The experience of a Bulgarian physician at Călăraşi DEH*

The hospital manager organized the interview with one of the Bulgarian anaesthetists at his workplace, the intensive care unit, together with his Romanian peers and the head of the unit to ensure a trusting and open atmosphere. The Romanian interpreter accompanied the Bulgarian doctor, as usual.

The doctor's working history in Romania began in September 2011. He learned about possible jobs in Romania from a Bulgarian colleague already working at Călăraşi DEH. A practising surgeon in Bulgaria, he began work as an anaesthetist in Romania (in addition, his wife is the neonatologist who was to enter into negotiations to join the Romanian hospital).

From the Bulgarian doctor's perspective, the main push to search for a job abroad was an economic one, given the very low level of income in Bulgaria. Another important factor was the highly bureaucratic relationship between Silistra Hospital and the health insurance company, which caused delays in physicians' payments at the Bulgarian hospital. His family was the main mitigating factor, as one of his children was yet to graduate from high school.

He considers his present job in Romania as a temporary to medium-term strategy because language is the main barrier to his career development in Romania, although he has started Romanian language classes. He might also consider applying for a job in western Europe where opportunities abound. Silistra has a surplus of anaesthetists, so foreign recruitment agencies from Germany, France, England, Denmark and Sweden are very active in the region. This is also a very promising resource for recruiting Bulgarian doctors to work in Romania.

The Bulgarian doctor is satisfied with his work and working conditions in Romania. He has had the opportunity to encounter a wide range of pathology, so his experience and knowledge have grown. He considers that he has built a solid team with his Romanian colleagues – both doctors and nurses – and shared their experiences and practice standards. He perceives himself as well integrated and accepted within the team. He would advertise jobs in Romania among his colleagues in Bulgaria.

Role of the EU

The case of Călăraşi DEH is not unique in Romania. Increased emigration of physicians and nurses began after 2007 when Romania joined the EU, and intensified after 2010 when government austerity measures to freeze all new recruitment to the public sector, together with 25% salary cuts, contributed to a real health workforce crisis in Romania (Galan et al., 2011). Almost all Romanian DEHs face significant staffing problems and several important medical specialties are not covered. The economic crisis and the lack of modern planning mechanisms for human resources for health are having a deep impact on continuity and quality of care, and on access to important health services, especially in the most deprived areas of Romania.

Recruitment of foreign physicians thus appears to offer one solution to overcome the shortage of doctors. Although evidence is not yet available from official data or other research studies, it is very likely that foreign doctors might also work in other hospitals in Romania. The Danube river border with Bulgaria continues for 470 km, passing alongside many other Romanian districts, so doctors from other regions of Bulgaria could also work in local Romanian hospitals.

The EU context facilitates diploma recognition to enable Bulgarian or Hungarian doctors to work in Romania. This is not the case for doctors from Serbia or Ukraine, however, as the EU does not fully recognize their diplomas. Physicians from the Republic of Moldova already work in Romanian hospitals, but their situation is different as they usually hold Romanian citizenship as well and complete their specialty training in Romanian medical universities (compulsory after 2007). Although the mobility of health care professionals across the Danube to Călăraşi DEH did not benefit from European funding, the right to free movement across borders as well as the system of diploma recognition within the EU facilitated the integration of Bulgarian physicians in the Romanian health care system.

Within the wider EU context, two cross-border projects to promote hospital collaboration across the Romanian–Hungarian border are currently under way, run by Arad DEH in Romania, within the Hungary–Romania Cross-border Co-operation Programme 2007–2013 (HURO, 2013). The "Improvement of telediagnostics network in the Csongrád-Arad region" project (HURO/0802/013) aims to offer efficient and safe solutions to health units lacking specialists in radiology and diagnostic equipment through telemedicine and a common patient database. The European Regional Development Fund provides 85% of the project's funding, with a global budget of €1.7 million. The "Cure without borders for the Criş Mureş region" project aims to improve standards of practice in emergency care by creating a common database for health care in the Arad and Békés districts in Romania and Hungary. The European Regional Development Fund also funds this project, with a global budget of €1.97 million. The implementation period for both projects is 2011–2013.

According to the classification of cross-border collaboration widely accepted in the literature (Glinos, 2011), both these projects cover a much wider range of collaboration activities, including movement of patients, exchange of services, exchange of health care professionals, and transfer and exchange of patient information. Since they only started in 2011 and are currently in progress, however, evaluation of their outputs and outcomes will occur after 2013.

EU-funded projects, as well as local initiatives such as the one in Călăraşi, might offer a solution for countries in eastern and south-eastern Europe to overcome the shortage of health care personnel and to secure equitable access for their populations to health services of high quality by building cooperation in the region. The South-eastern Europe Health Network has established another promising scheme for regional cooperation by setting up a new Regional Health Development Centre for Health Human Resources at Kishinev in the Republic of Moldova. The Centre's aims are to build a well-trained health workforce in south-eastern Europe and to create mechanisms to retain and motivate physicians and nurses to practise in their countries of origin.

Future outlook

For the general manager of Călăraşi DEH, attracting physicians from Bulgaria to work at the hospital is a medium- or long-term strategy to overcome the shortage of physicians in the national health care system. This is a revealing perspective and raises the question of whether there might be scope for more official collaboration between the two hospitals. Although not collaborating in a formal or structural way, the two hospitals are de facto engaged in exchanges as doctors from Silistra work at Călăraşi and Silistra Hospital provides maternity care to Romanian women living in the border region. Commuting Bulgarian doctors act as unofficial communicators between the two organizations and it is conceivable that contact may increase as cross-border recruitment continues and even expands over the years. Since they partially share the same medical workforce, and with no obvious end in sight to the staffing shortages in Romania, it could benefit the two hospitals to communicate on a more official level.

Virtually all the posts of the 200 or so health professionals who left Călăraşi DEH in 2010–2011 have remained vacant. While the Bulgarian doctors ensure the continuity of an essential aspect of hospital services, their part-time contracts do not amount to a full-time equivalent. A freeze on filling vacancies in the public service until a ratio of 7:1 is reached, including in all publicly financed and run hospitals, is one of the harsh measures taken by the government to counteract the effects of the economic crisis in 2009. This means that only one replacement can be hired for every seven health professionals lost. Călăraşi DEH also cannot remove the vacant positions because this could mean that it loses its classification as a district hospital.

Romanian physicians are in short supply almost everywhere in Romania, with the exception of the big cities with medical universities. Since hospitals can hire both Romanian and EU doctors under the same legal conditions, it is often easier to find physicians from abroad keen to work in Romania, despite the lengthy verification and registration procedures this entails. This reflects the constraints that Călăraşi DEH and other Romanian hospitals face and is one of the reasons district health authorities call for greater autonomy from central decision-making, especially concerning human resources management and establishment of hospital structures. Until that happens, Călăraşi DEH seems to have no option but to fill vacancies by contracting doctors from across the border, giving rise to the paradox that in times of economic crisis a Romanian employer is forced to import workforce from abroad.

Conclusion

It would be very interesting to evaluate the impact of health care professionals' mobility on the Romanian health care system. One direct financial impact as defined in the literature (Baeten, 2011), for example, is on the administrative burden of Călăraşi DEH: the time and effort spent on solving the difficulties of licensing foreign physicians to practise in Romania (Interview 3). Unfortunately, details of these costs are not available.

The hospital manager was confident that patient access to health care services has increased as a result of the cross-border collaboration, leading to fewer referrals to hospitals in Bucharest for common surgical interventions. Patient mobility, as well as health care worker mobility, means that the geographical barrier posed by the Danube river border is not perceived as an issue. Physicians at Silistra Hospital offer their services to Romanian women living south of the Danube who deliver in Bulgaria because it is closer than Călăraşi DEH. Another important impact on quality of care was the adoption of new standards of practice introduced by the foreign doctors to Romania.

Interviewees called for greater decision-making authority at the district level, arguing that cross-border mobility should be a temporary solution to overcome Călăraşi DEH's lack of independence in matters of human resources management and hospital structure. All the health reforms under debate in the late 2000s and early 2010s proposed to grant hospitals significantly more room for negotiation in these areas, but have not yet been implemented in mid-2013. Cross-border mobility adds value to improved hospital governance by moving towards autonomy. Autonomous hospitals can more easily attract (human) resources to fill existing gaps, as the hospital management has more discretion in using its management tools, under different legal arrangements.

Despite more and more warning signals about the deepening shortage of health personnel in the Romanian health system, the situation had worsened by 2013. One might conclude that most of the DEHs in Romania could adopt the solution found by Călăraşi DEH, although hospitals in border regions may be at an advantage in terms of attracting skilled health professionals from neighbouring countries. Călăraşi's example of overcoming the language barrier may also create awareness of the need for another staff role in the Romanian health system: the interpreter.

References

Baeten R (2011). Past impacts of cross-border health care. In: Wismar M, Palm W, Figueras J, Ernst K and Van Ginneken E, eds. *Cross-border health care in the European Union: mapping and analysing practices and policies.* Copenhagen, WHO Regional Office for Europe on behalf of the European Observatory on Health Systems and Policies (Observatory Studies Series, No. 22: 255–87; www.euro.who.int/__data/assets/pdf_file/0004/135994/e94875.pdf, accessed 1 July 2013).

Călăraşi District Council (2012). Informatii generale despre Călăraşi [General information about Călăraşi] [web site]. Călăraşi, Consiliul Judetean Calarasi (www.calarasi.ro/ro/, accessed 1 July 2013).

Galan A, Olsavszky V, Vlădescu C (2011). Emergent challenge of health professional emigration: Romania's accession to the European Union. In: Wismar M, Maier CB, Glinos IA, Dussault G, Figueras J, eds. *Health professional mobility and health systems: evidence from 17 European countries.* Copenhagen, WHO Regional Office for Europe on behalf of the European Observatory on Health Systems and Policies (Observatory Studies Series, No. 23: 449–77; www.euro.who.int/__data/assets/pdf_file/0017/152324/e95812.pdf, accessed 2 July 2013).

Glinos IA (2011). Cross-border collaboration. In: Wismar M, Palm W, Figueras J, Ernst K and Van Ginneken E, eds. *Cross-border health care in the European Union: mapping and analysing practices and policies.* Copenhagen, WHO Regional Office for Europe on behalf of the European Observatory on Health Systems and Policies (Observatory Studies Series, No. 22: 217–54; www.euro.who.int/__data/assets/pdf_file/0004/135994/e94875.pdf, accessed 20 December 2012).

HURO (2013). Hungary–Romania Cross-border Co-operation Programme 2007–2013 [web site]. Budapest, VÁTI Nonprofit Kft (www.huro-cbc.eu/en/, accessed 3 July 2013).

Ministry of Health (2011). *Health Statistics Yearbook.* Bucharest, Ministry of Health.

National Institute of Statistics (2010). Health Units Activity. Bucharest, Institutul National de Statistica.

Novinite (2011). Bulgarian doctors go abroad for better pay, union says. *BalkanInsight*, 27 January (www.balkaninsight.com/en/article/bulgarian-doctors-go-abroad-for-better-pay-union-says, accessed 2 July 2013).

Stroe M (2011). Călăraşi District Council took over the hospital from Budeşti. *Obiectiv*, 130, April (www.obiectiv-online.ro/consiliul_judetean_calarasi_a_preluat_spitalul_din.html, accessed 20 January 2012).

Vlădescu C, Scîntee G, Olsavszky V, Allin S, Mladovsky P (2008). Romania: Health system review. *Health Systems in Transition*, 10(3): 1–172 (www.euro.who.int/__data/assets/pdf_file/0008/95165/E91689.pdf, accessed 1 July 2013).

WHO (2011). *Technical Meeting Report on Health Workforce Retention in countries of the South-eastern Europe Health Network.* Copenhagen, WHO Regional Office for Europe (www.euro.who.int/__data/assets/pdf_file/0018/152271/e95775.pdf, accessed 1 July 2013).

Annex 8.1 Interviews conducted

Number	Date	Interviewee	Institution
Interview 1	15 December 2011	Dr Corina Sebe, Executive Director	Călăraşi DPHD
Interview 2	15 December 2011	Dr Camelia Truica, Head of Health Status Evaluation and Health Promotion Department	Călăraşi DPHD
Interview 3	15 December 2011	Dr Victor Verinceanu, General Manager	Călăraşi DEH
Interview 4	15 December 2011	Dr Mariana Chiru, Head of Intensive Care Unit	Călăraşi DEH
Interview 5	15 December 2011	Bulgarian doctor	Călăraşi DEH

One hospital for the border region: building the new Cerdanya Hospital (Spain–France)

José Miguel Sanjuán and Joan Gil

Introduction

The cross-border Cerdanya Hospital project was the first European initiative to build a new facility aimed at providing health care services to patients from two different national health systems (France and Catalonia/Spain), bringing together patients, professionals, medical protocols, administrative procedures and laws from countries with deep institutional differences. This chapter describes and analyses the definition and construction stages of Cerdanya Hospital as a cross-border health care facility from its inception. It shows how the hospital has become a tool for fostering territorial cohesion, recognizing that part of its success results from a long history of political and institutional collaboration among stakeholders in the territory. The authors believe that Cerdanya Hospital represents a natural experiment worth further study, particularly into the wide array of problems and difficulties encountered when dealing with the construction of complex supranational institutions and organizations working at the European level.

Methodology

The authors collected data in three different stages during 2010 and 2011 to complete the study. They first searched all relevant documentation regarding the process of creating Cerdanya Hospital and the different institutions and stakeholders involved. They also performed a literature review, including local and regional newspapers mentioning Cerdanya Hospital and grey literature such as annual reports of the institutions involved in the process. To support this information they held several interviews with the general manager of Puigcerdà Hospital to obtain first-hand information on the new hospital's creation.

They then selected key stakeholders in order to capture the particularities of the actors involved and conducted semi-structured interviews, which they recorded. After the interviews, they asked respondents to cite other potential key actors; this allowed them to contact further stakeholders (see Annex 9.1 for interview details). The authors conducted all interviews face to face at the interviewee's place of work, whether on the Catalan or the French side. The interviews lasted between two and three hours and took place mainly in Catalan but also in Spanish.

The border region and health care context

Geography

Cerdanya ("Cerdaña" in Spanish; "Cerdagne" in French) is an isolated valley with a large, high plateau set in the mountainous area of the Pyrenees. The region is divided into Upper Cerdanya (the northern part) in France and Lower Cerdanya (the southern part) on the Spanish side of the border (Map 9.1). Historically, the entire territory of Cerdanya was one of the counties of Catalonia and the split occurred as a result of the Treaty of the Pyrenees of 1659.

Today Lower Cerdanya (henceforth Cerdanya) is a Catalan county covering an area of 546.6 km^2 with a population of more than 18 500 inhabitants – a density of 33.9 inhabitants/km^2. The municipality of Puigcerdà, the county's capital since the twelfth century when it replaced Hix (now Bourg-Madame in France), has a population of more than 8 700 inhabitants: 47% of the whole county's population. Puigcerdà City Council is the largest in the valley and one of the most important in the Pyrenees. The area's main economic activity is tourism (mostly winter sports), with some services and livestock. Average gross domestic product (GDP) per capita in Cerdanya was €29 300 in 2006, 7.4% higher than that of Catalonia as a whole (Idescat, 2010). Puigcerdà Hospital is the most important employer in the region.

The French side, Upper Cerdanya, is part of the Pyrénées-Orientales department in the Languedoc-Roussillon region, with a population of 14 966 inhabitants within 540 km^2. Its most important municipalities are Font-Romeu-Odeillo-Via, Osséja (which has an important sanatorium), Bourg-Madame and Saillagose. Again, its main economic activity relies on the tourism sector, although the dairy industry is also important. Sanatoria, mostly built in the latter half of the nineteenth century and linked to the treatment of tuberculosis, have traditionally been another important source of income for the area. Over time many of these have been replaced by health spas as a result of the rise of so-called "health tourism", but the tradition of convalescence continues as modern-day recovery centres have a strong presence in the region.

Map 9.1. *Upper and Lower Cerdanya*

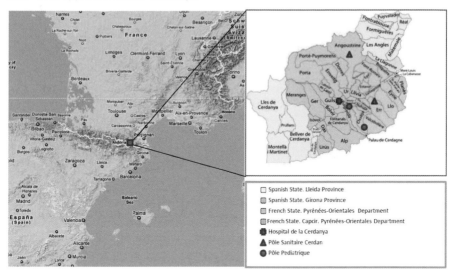

Source: Authors' elaboration based on figures extracted from Google Maps and i-Cerdanya.info.

GDP per capita on the French and Catalan sides of the border has evolved differently over the last two decades (Table 9.1). Interestingly, despite a lack of natural barriers, the historical artificial border between the two countries has separated the two communities for centuries, making them develop in different directions (Salvat et al., 1997). While these differences have remained during recent decades despite European integration, the fact that a significant proportion of the French population of Cerdanya speaks Catalan[1] has contributed to reinforcing political contacts among local stakeholders. These close ties have meant, for example, that some children from Puigcerdà go to school in neighbouring Bourg-Madame, citizens of Bourg-Madame visit Puigcerdà to participate in sports, and so on.

Table 9.1. *GDP per capita (euros), 1997–2008*

Area	1997	Index[a]	2008	Index
European Union	16 200	100	25 100	100
France	21 000	130	30 400	121
Pyrénées-Orientales	15 500	96	22 700	90
Catalonia	15 700	97	27 900	111
Girona[b]	16 100	99	27 200	108

Source: Eurostat data on GDP per inhabitant at current market prices by Nomenclature of Territorial Units for Statistics (NUTS) level 3 region.
Note: a Index European Union = 100, b Girona includes Catalan Cerdanya.

---

1   According to the Catalan government, 65% of the population of Upper Cerdanya understands Catalan, although this percentage decreases to around 50% among those aged 15 to 29. In contrast, Catalan is understood by 94.6% of the population across the border in Catalonia.

In 1991 the entire Cerdanya valley became part of the Pyrenees–Mediterranean Euroregion, which initially included Catalonia and the French regions of Languedoc-Roussillon and Midi-Pyrénées. In 2004 two more Spanish regions joined: Aragon and the Balearic Islands.

Health care system and patient flows

A duality affects the whole Cerdanya border region. As well as the hospital at Puigcerdà the next closest Catalan hospital is in Manresa, which is 100 km to the south and connected by well-maintained main roads. The French side, however, is relatively isolated. Prades, which has a small health centre, is 59 km away, while the hospital at Perpignan (capital of the Pyrénées-Orientales department) is 103 km away, but the road is sinuous and the heavy weather conditions in winter can result in a lengthy trip or even an impassable route. As a result the French population began to use services provided by Puigcerdà Hospital.

Three types of health care institution coexist across the region: French family doctors, French recovery centres and Puigcerdà Hospital. On the French side family doctors are independent professionals operating privately under market conditions. The 14 public and private health centres (see Annex 9.2) specialize in recovery care and continuous assistance; these are highly subsidized, following either the former concept of the "Participant au Service Public Hospitalier" model, for which they receive a fixed yearly amount, or the "Objectif Quantifié National" model, for which they receive funding depending on the number of patients treated. A seemingly high rate of underutilization characterizes these centres, which had over 800 beds among them in 2003.

On the Catalan side the main health care provider is Puigcerdà Hospital, operated by a private foundation that is part of the Xarxa Hospitalària d'Utilització Pública (the public hospital network), overseen by the Catalan Health Service. Unusually, the mayor of Puigcerdà is the president of the foundation and is involved in the management of the hospital. Puigcerdà Hospital Foundation provides three types of service: primary care (via the health centres of Puigcerdà and Bellver), hospital care (with 30 acute care beds, 19 outpatient beds, 2 operating rooms and 1 delivery room) and a skilled nursing home (with 130 beds for long- and medium-term stays). It is the most important organization in Cerdanya in economic terms.

It is important to note that while Catalan health policy relies on a model of local hospital networks, in France hospitals are more geographically concentrated with networks of thematic health clusters and with heavy reliance on patient transport. The practice of offering long recovery periods in specialized centres is also more widespread in France (Harant, 2006; Bourret and Tort i Bardolet, 2003).

To give an idea of the magnitude of patient flows, between 2007 and 2011 Puigcerdà Hospital treated a total of 7401 French patients (Table 9.2). Of those, about 48% were outpatients, 40% emergency cases, 8% in receipt of other hospital services and 3% maternity patients. French payments represented roughly 5% of the Catalan hospital's total revenue in 2008 (last information available).

Table 9.2. *French patients admitted to Puigcerdà Hospital, 2007–2011*

Department	2007	2008	2009	2010	2011
Outpatients	696	586	777	814	676
Emergency	491	502	772	654	568
Other hospital services	114	104	116	161	132
Maternity	51	50	41	58	38

Source: data provided by Puigcerdà Hospital.

Evolution of the new hospital: a chronological perspective

Background: 1980s to 2002

The idea of building a new cross-border hospital dates back to the 1980s. It arose partly in response to the need of the population of Upper Cerdanya to have access to certain health services (including birth and emergency care) when, especially under adverse weather conditions, the time taken to reach the nearest French hospital in Perpignan could cause or exacerbate serious health problems. Although Puigcerdà Hospital was easily accessible, at the beginning of the 1990s visits from French patients were few, as it seems cultural barriers and distrust of the Catalan/Spanish health system meant that only the most severe cases sought assistance at the hospital.

Although according to several sources an initial draft of a cross-border hospital proposal developed by the Catalan administration existed, nobody took the project seriously until the mid-1990s. The relationship between the manager of Puigcerdà Hospital at that time and the mayor of Puigcerdà from 1995 to 2003, who was also a doctor at Puigcerdà Hospital (and who went on to become minister of governance and public administration of the Catalan government in 2003–2006), helped to resurrect the old idea. They observed an increase in the number of visits by French patients to the hospital, although without reimbursement from French insurance funds (Glinos and Baeten, 2006). Between 1997 and 2002 the number of French patients hospitalized or admitted for emergency care at Puigcerdà almost tripled (from 68 to 190), while payment remained unsettled in 50% of cases (Tobar Pascual, 2003).

The stakeholders solved this problem by setting up an agreement in 2002 between Puigcerdà Hospital, Perpignan Hospital and Languedoc-Roussillon Regional Health Agency to organize reimbursement for the provision of emergency services to French patients retrospectively from 2001. A second agreement with the same actors followed in 2003, precisely regulating procedures for emergency and birth care at Puigcerdà Hospital. This evolved satisfactorily over time as French doctors and patients gained confidence in the Catalan health system. For instance, in obstetrics assistance evolved from visits covering the last weeks of pregnancy to broader monitoring of the patient (currently following up future mothers from the seventh month) (Interview 2).

According to one interviewee, these agreements were possible because of the existence of previous political, economic and personal links across the border, especially among the local mayors, which facilitated reconsideration of the old project (Interview 8). In fact, the hospital was not the first or only cross-border initiative undertaken in the area: in 1993 parties on both sides drew up an agreement to share a sewage treatment plant, which is still operational. A previous agreement managed by mayors from France and Spain regulating the international water channel of Cerdanya even dates back to 1866. According to the mayor of Bourg-Madame there have been talks about setting up a cross-border secondary school based in Bourg-Madame, and a project to create a cross-border slaughterhouse in Ur (on the French side) (Interview 9). A recent ambitious project aims to teach graduate odontology courses within Puigcerdà Hospital jointly with the Universities of Vic and Paul Sabatier of Toulouse, sharing students between Toulouse and Puigcerdà (Interview 7). The ultimate objective of these extended cross-border collaborations is to transform the area to avoid the region's constant loss of human capital and high dependence on the tourism sector.

First steps: 2002–2003

In 2002 the mayors of Puigcerdà and Bourg-Madame jointly initiated the first moves to gain the French government's support for the project to build a cross-border hospital. With the help of a local French member of parliament they went to Paris to contact a well-placed politician in the cabinet of the French Ministry of Solidarity and Social Cohesion, Ministry of Health and Ministry of Social Affairs – a native of the region and supporter of regional integration, as well as a key figure in the Languedoc-Roussillon Regional Health Agency. Together they agreed the idea of (partially) financing the future cross-border hospital with funding from the European Regional Development Fund (ERDF).

At the same time the presidents of the Catalan government and Languedoc-Roussillon signed a letter of intent to prepare a feasibility study for a new cross-border hospital in Cerdanya. The feasibility project was the result of an agreement between the government of Catalonia, the Languedoc-Roussillon Regional Health Agency, the Conseil Régional du Languedoc-Roussillon, the Conseil Général des Pyrénnées-Orientales and the Puigcerdà Hospital Foundation. The study drew four main conclusions (Rodríguez and Conill, 2003).

- The project would be viable if the administrative agencies in charge of planning and funding public health (the Languedoc-Roussillon Regional Health Agency and Catalan Health Service) co-owned the new cross-border hospital. A juridical formula should be found to enable this.

- The new hospital should replace the existing Puigcerdà Hospital and offer assistance to acute patients across the whole Cerdanya region.

- It should be located in Puigcerdà and integrate the current health networks of the two different public administrations.

- It should also respect the cultural and health particularities of both countries.[2]

Once the feasibility report confirmed the project's viability and gave general outlines, responsibility passed to the institutions in charge of developing it: the Catalan Health Service and Languedoc-Roussillon Regional Health Agency. According to the current operations director of the Pyrenees Health Region, the project was a courageous one and its initial success resulted from its relevance to larger political initiatives in France and Catalonia (Interview 4). On the Catalan side, for instance, the government's policy of creating networks of local hospitals (as with the health regions of the Alt Pirineu i Aran: Vall de Aran in 1985, Seu de Urgell in 1992 and Pallars in 1993) dates from the 1980s. In consequence, the idea of a new hospital financed by European funds to replace the one dating from the seventeenth century perfectly fits within this policy. On the French side, the project would offer a better health service to the isolated Upper Cerdanya, and the decision to fund a new hospital also occurred in the middle of an initiative to restructure the French health care sector.

Creating agreement: 2004–2010

From 2004 to 2007 the two administrations entered a period of negotiation. An unparalleled number of local, regional and national elections slowed the process as the individual actors involved in the discussions changed frequently, but in July 2007 the French and Catalan health ministries signed an agreement to fund Cerdanya Hospital. In March 2009 ERDF funding of €18.6 million

---

2   Data from the authors' conversations with X. Conill, co-author of the feasibility study (Interview 3).

was approved through the POCTEFA 2007–2013 programme, which finances economic and social integration of the cross-border regions of Spain, France and Andorra through ERDF funds amounting to €168 million (POCTEFA, 2008).

Once both parties agreed the general outline of the project and its funding, the process of negotiating the statutes of the new hospital lasted until the spring of 2010 (BOE, 2011; Box 9.1). Although negotiations took place mainly between the Catalan Health Service and the Languedoc-Roussillon Regional Health Agency, the central governments of Barcelona, Madrid and Paris had to make or ratify some of the decisions.

Box 9.1. *Setting up EGTC Cerdanya Hospital*

EGTC Cerdanya Hospital – the largest EGTC constituted to date – is the legal instrument adopted to manage the new cross-border hospital (BOE, 2011; European Commission, 2011). Created on 26 April 2010, it involves the Catalan government on the Spanish side and the Languedoc-Roussillon Regional Health Agency, national health insurance fund Caisse nationale de l'assurance maladie des travailleurs salariés (CNAMTS) and French Ministry of Health on the French side.

The EGTC replaced the Fundació Privada Hospital Transfronterer de la Cerdanya, which had been in charge of the construction of the hospital since 2006. The main reason for its adoption was the Treaty of Bayonne, by which the French and Spanish administrations are bound, which states that they cannot manage foreign funds and that only institutions at the same level can sign agreements.[3] The EGTC formula was the optimal juridical solution to overcome such limitations. In addition, the new instrument can receive and manage ERDF funds, govern the hospital and bring together foreign institutions at different levels.

From the beginning EGTC Cerdanya Hospital was set up to construct and manage the new hospital within the jurisdiction of European law, using Spanish law when the broader approach was not applicable. It is also responsible for purchasing health services from providers in both countries. EGTC Cerdanya Hospital is subject to the accounting rules and supervisory bodies of Spain, which will transfer the information to their equivalents in France. It has four governing bodies.

- The board of directors approves and supervises the management of EGTC Cerdanya Hospital, sets policy and appoints the executive commission. It comprises 14 members: eight from Catalonia, elected by the Catalan health minister, and six from France, elected by the Languedoc-Roussillon Regional Health Agency. Catalan members include the mayor of Puigcerdà and the president of the county council, a local administrative body grouping the county's mayors. French members include four representatives of the

---

3 Thus, for example, city councils can sign agreements with other city councils but not with regional bodies.

French government, the director of the Languedoc-Roussillon Regional Health Agency and a representative of CNAMTS. The director of Cerdanya Hospital is also a (non-voting) member of the board. Every two years the presidency and vice-presidency alternate between the two countries (Catalonia currently holds the presidency and France the vice-presidency). The board takes its decisions based on a simple majority of voting members.

- The executive commission is the purchasing body, which deals with day-to-day decision-making, advises the board of directors and decides the outline of EGTC Cerdanya Hospital management. It comprises five representatives: three from Catalonia and two from France.

- The consultative body or advisory council is composed of local mayors and relevant stakeholders. It scrutinizes the decisions taken by the board of directors and its role is to express its opinion, although without voting rights. It comprises 14 members: eight from the Catalan and six from the French side.

- The director of EGTC Cerdanya Hospital, appointed by the board of directors as advised by the executive commission, acts as CEO, applying the decisions of the board and executive commission.

Source: BOE, 2011.

Three main critical issues appeared during the negotiation phase (Interview 4).

- A new instrument, the European Grouping of Territorial Cooperation Hospital de la Cerdanya (EGTC Cerdanya Hospital), became the governing body of the new hospital. It represented both administrations but the French government did not agree to share responsibility with a regional government, wanting an agreement between Spain and France, not between Catalonia and France. Eventually the Spanish Ministry of Health became involved in the project, thus solving the problem.

- The next issue concerned responsibility for funding the day-to-day costs of Cerdanya Hospital. The negotiations ended in an agreement that the French side would finance 40% and the Catalan side 60% during the first five years (2012–2017), following which a new agreement should take into account the number and proportion of French patients served by the new hospital. The underlying purpose of this arrangement was to unify prices, under the principle that the same tariff should apply for every patient, whether paid by the Catalan Health Service or the Languedoc-Roussillon Regional Health Agency.

- Another initial proposal was that the governing body would include local mayors, an idea grounded in an established tradition in Catalonia that favours close monitoring of the provision of certain public services by local politicians. The Catalan government was in favour of this move but the French government disagreed. The negotiations ended with the creation of a "consultative body", which included local politicians, within the EGTC.

In parallel, the French government had to overcome another important political issue. Upper Cerdanya contained a network of health centres focused mainly on the recovery of patients with respiratory illnesses. This network had become unsustainable over time, and in the 2000s the French government aimed to rationalize the sector, forcing the centres to collaborate and optimize resources. The government thus faced the difficulty of explaining to its constituents the decision to close local recovery centres while funding a new hospital in Catalan Cerdanya.

To help rationalize the region's resources a new cross-border care project emerged, initially put forward by the feasibility study. This entailed the creation of two new health facilities on the French side of the border – a "pôle gériatrique" (geriatric health centre) in Err and a "pôle pédiatrique" (paediatric health centre) in Bourg-Madame – as a way of rationalizing the surplus of French health care professionals by integrating some of the French recovery centres into the orbit of the services needed for Cerdanya Hospital.[4] The new health centres offer services not provided by the hospital: long-, medium- and short-term geriatric and paediatric care (Interviews 5 and 6). Table 9.3 summarizes the provisional investment funding sources for each facility.

Table 9.3. *Provisional investment plan*

Facility	Funding		Investment (€ million)	Proportion (%)	Total (€ million)
Cerdanya Hospital	France		4.7	16	
	Catalonia		7.4	24	30.7
	ERDF		18.6	60	
Geriatric health centre	EGTC Cerdanya Hospital	France	1.1	8	
		Catalonia	0.5	4	
	Local recovery centres		9.5	67	14.1
	ERDF		3.0	21	
Paediatric health centre	France		0.4	4	
	Catalonia		0.19	2	
	Local recovery centres		8.2	82	10
	ERDF		1.2	12	

Source: Boix, 2011 (figures for the health centres are forecasts).

---

4 These health centres will legally take the form of a "groupement de coopération sanitaire", a legal instrument facilitating cooperation between private and public health professionals and institutions.

The internal structure of the health centres is still under consideration, with the involvement of the Languedoc-Roussillon Regional Health Agency and Catalan Health Service. One of the first steps will be the creation of a mobile geriatric health care team to lend support to Cerdanya Hospital, composed of French and Catalan staff. The next stage will probably be to unify criteria, establishing a joint tariff and an information technology system that supports both the hospital and the health centres.

These broader ideas of care delivery show how both administrations have shifted their perspectives, and since 2007–2008 have started to talk of a wider territorial project instead of just the setting up of a new hospital. The success of the two health centres and of Cerdanya Hospital will depend on their managing to attract patients who currently seek health care outside the valley.

Current status of Cerdanya Hospital

Building work on the new hospital started in 2008 and was close to completion in 2012. The hospital expects to begin activity in 2013. It will have 64 beds, 11 day hospital places, 13 emergency beds, 13 dialysis stations, 4 operating rooms and an MRI scanner. Of the €31 million investment (see Table 9.3), the total cost of equipment is forecast to be €10 million, of which €3 million is earmarked for information technology (Actualitat la Cerdanya, 2012). The hospital plans to employ 201 professional staff members (Table 9.4). This is a rise of 46% on personnel numbers at Puigcerdà Hospital; in particular, the number of doctors will rise from 36 to 50 and the number of nurses and midwives from 43 to 58 (Fundació Privada Hospital de Puigcerdà, 2010; Boix, 2011).[5]

Table 9.4. *Staff numbers forecast at Cerdanya Hospital (initial stage)*

Role	Number
Doctor	50
Nurse/midwife	58
Technical personnel	42
Management – administration – patient care	30
Other staff	21
Total	**201**

Source: Boix, 2011.

---

5   The most recent information provided to the authors is that EGTC Cerdanya Hospital, the governing body of the new hospital, will purchase the necessary health services mainly from those institutions available within the region (Puigcerdà Hospital, Perpignan Hospital, and so on).

The annual budget of Cerdanya Hospital will amount to about €17.5 million (Table 9.5). This must provide the necessary financial means for the new hospital to start its cross-border care activities, which both administrations will examine after the first five years. In order to become viable, the new hospital needs to attract, during this initial period, about 5500 hospital admissions from Upper Cerdanya that currently visit other French health centres for treatment.

Table 9.5. *Estimated operating costs of Cerdanya Hospital*

Category	Cost (€ million)
Purchasing	3.845
Outsourcing services	1.350
Taxes	0.040
Human resources	10.130
Financial expenses	0.025
Exceptional expenses	0.025
Depreciation and amortization	2.000
Total	**17.415**

Source: Boix, 2011.

Needs and incentives

The necessity that sparked the creation of Cerdanya Hospital was local need: French patients needed faster access to hospital services, since under certain circumstances they were at considerable risk. Upper Cerdanya's low population density and lack of large villages meant that the region could not build a new local hospital under the French government's health policy, which promoted large geographically concentrated hospitals. On the Catalan side, even taking into account the important floating population associated with tourism in the area (some years reaching more than 100 000 people) and the Catalan policy of small networked hospitals, investment in a new health care facility was not a priority because a local hospital already existed. Nevertheless, the old Puigcerdà Hospital could not accommodate the expansion of services resulting from increased numbers of French patients, so the area needed a new hospital, ideally with updated and improved facilities to continue to attract more cross-border patients.

The institutions involved thus began to collaborate primarily because, even though both sides needed improved local hospital facilities, they could not undertake the cross-border health care project independently. As a result they established a win–win relationship. A project of this scale inevitably at some point develops its own momentum: this section analyses each institution's internal incentives to collaborate, the obstacles that arose and the solutions developed to overcome them.

For Puigcerdà Hospital the collaboration offered opportunities to expand its activities and gain a new and modern hospital, to incorporate experienced French professionals into an already established team, and to rethink the services the hospital should provide (Interviews 1 and 2). For Puigcerdà City Council the new hospital was a chance to diversify the city's economic activity by expanding a sector with high added value. As a result the staff of both organizations were deeply involved in the project and prepared themselves over the seven years of its development to face the challenges that becoming part of the new cross-border hospital would entail, by learning French or dealing with the legal and administrative problems of the management of the cross-border collaboration. This may also explain why the mayors of Puigcerdà and Bourg-Madame did not accept the new de facto situation when they lost control of the project around 2004 (when the Catalan and French governments took over). The words of the current mayor of Puigcerdà – "We do not want the result of moving the hospital one kilometre away to be that the management is hundreds of kilometres away" (Interview 7) – reflect the desire to maintain control over an institution that had always been managed locally. Inclusion of local governments in the consultative body of EGTC Cerdanya Hospital was a way of calming the waters, for the moment.

Conversely, the 2002 agreement solved the French government's specific problems with the delivery of health services in Upper Cerdanya. Analysis of the information provided suggests that an additional incentive for the French side to participate in the cross-border hospital project was that it could contribute to solving the problem of their seemingly underused recovery centres. Transforming them into the two new geriatric and paediatric health centres would integrate them into a larger cross-border area of service provision. Although the 2003 feasibility study first considered this option, it did not take shape until 2008 and is still being refined.

The delay suffered by the new hospital seems to be a consequence of dealing with multiple stakeholders, as is the case in Upper Cerdanya where there are many little villages. The Joseph Sauvy Centre led the process of establishing the geriatric health centre on the French side, forming a partnership with the Centre des Escaldes and EGTC Cerdanya Hospital, mainly because it is part of a larger association with 26 health centres in the department. The two partner recovery centres see the project as a way to ensure their survival and remain in the region.

It is also noteworthy that, according to one interviewee, the ultimate objective of the extended regional collaboration is to transform the territory to avoid the loss of human capital and high dependence on the tourism sector (Interview 7).

Future outlook: problems and solutions

To understand how Cerdanya Hospital will evolve in the future it is necessary to consider the problems encountered during its inception as these have shaped its subsequent development. Fundamentally, the establishment of the cross-border hospital means that three key groups of actors who previously had very little interaction will suddenly need to start cooperating closely. The relationships within and between these groups will change as they have to adopt new roles (Figs. 9.1 and 9.2).

EGTC Cerdanya Hospital will become the main supplier of health services in the territory, financed by the French and Catalan governments (see Table 9.2). Puigcerdà Hospital Foundation will transform, shifting its activity to the new Cerdanya Hospital. Puigcerdà City Council, which had a high degree of control over the management of the old Puigcerdà Hospital, will lose part of this influence over the new hospital to the Catalan Health Service and Languedoc-Roussillon Regional Health Agency. Some of the French recovery centres in Upper Cerdanya will need to convert their activities to support the region's new geriatric and paediatric health centres. Finally, the French family doctors will have to deal with a new health system context that could reduce their workload.

All these different stakeholders will have to establish new formal and informal relationships as interaction becomes the norm. The following subsections analyse issues that have arisen and consider some of the strategies developed to overcome this potentially conflictive situation and create equilibrium between the various parties.

Patients and health professionals

Patients are the cornerstone that will make the cross-border collaboration project viable. Catalan patients will see few differences at Cerdanya Hospital as the staff will initially consist mainly of local professionals. French patients, on the other hand, will face significant changes, including the need to opt out of their own health system (Interviews 5 and 6), which may well give rise to natural concerns. Doubts may also develop from the uncertainties associated with the cross-border hospital project; for example, will patients be able to choose which hospital they attend, and will they have the choice of going to Prades instead of Puigcerdà if they call an ambulance? French patients are used to having a great degree of freedom to choose their health care provider, so it is essential for the new hospital to "win them over". Some of the local population may remember that wealthy Catalan patients historically chose to visit French health centres rather than the local hospital when they encountered a medical problem;

Fig. 9.1. *Key stakeholders before establishment of Cerdanya Hospital*

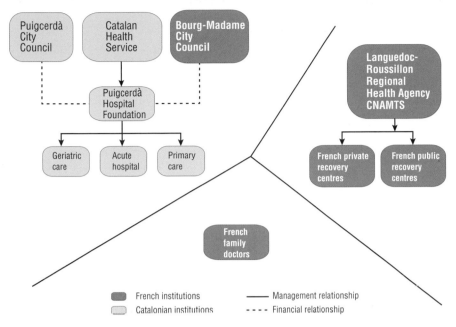

Source: Authors' compilation based on stakeholder interviews.

Fig. 9.2. *Key stakeholders once Cerdanya Hospital is operational*

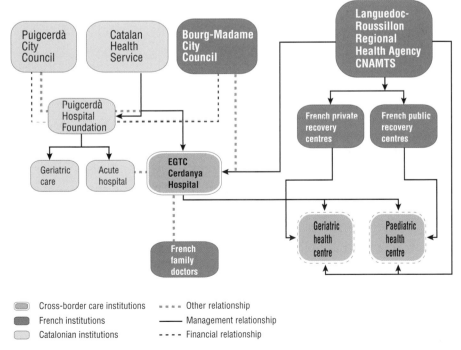

Source: Authors' compilation based on stakeholder interviews.

this may also exacerbate such concerns and make acceptance of the reverse situation where French patients have to seek health care in Catalonia difficult (Interviews 5 and 6).

The key to attracting French patients to Cerdanya Hospital is clear: the hospital's future success, in the opinion of both French and Catalan managers, depends on the recruitment of personnel from both countries. The underlying idea, therefore, is not to simply close Puigcerdà Hospital and open a new version of it, but to create a real cross-border health facility. To accomplish this objective, from the very beginning a significant proportion of the staff (not only doctors but all personnel) must come from the French side (Interviews 1, 2, 3, 5, 6 and 10). This policy serves a further purpose: Cerdanya Hospital will offer employment opportunities for French professionals who wish to work within the framework of the EGTC. The new hospital needs to attract a certain number of admissions from the territory in the first five years, as well as admissions from the non-resident floating population, to ensure viability.

This strategy relies on understanding the cultural differences between the French and Spanish health care systems (Interview 4). For instance, in France family doctors providing primary care closely assist patients (recommending, for instance, when they should go to hospital or which hospital they should attend), while in Spain general practitioners (GPs) do not follow up with the patient throughout the process. Patients in France also spend longer in hospital, while the Spanish health care system tends to favour shorter stays using home care services as an alternative. Other minor differences include the more formal or polite relationship French patients and doctors are used to, compared to a more direct form of contact in Spain. If the hospital applies Spanish standards rigidly the authors are inclined to believe that French patients could be somewhat disappointed with the service. In addition, Cerdanya Hospital will need to gain the confidence of French patients without interfering with the usual practice of the French doctors it needs to refer those patients to its services; this means that the hospital must provide the medical tests and services not available on the French side to avoid competition with French health professionals. Another potential problem not mentioned by the stakeholders could be dealing with differences in patients' rights, as Spanish law gives patients legal rights vis-à-vis their medical doctor whereas French patients have quasi-legal rights (Nys and Goffin, 2011).

The construction of Cerdanya Hospital and probable diminution or closure of facilities in French recovery centres could appear to be moving good jobs from France to Catalonia, which might endanger the likelihood of French health professionals collaborating in the project. Moreover, potential resistance by some French professionals "could emerge in case of working in Spain if they consider it might mean a loss of social rights" (Interview 10). Trade unions are particularly concerned with how the new hospital would absorb French staff, especially when social security contributions by French workers are about double those of their Catalan counterparts. Similarly, wage differences are considerable, especially in the early stages for certain professions, favouring French workers. This could cause a problem for recruitment and retention and infringe EC regulations;[6] trade unions defend the position that health professionals should not accept a dual wage scale.

Medical protocols

Both sides recognized, perhaps surprisingly, that unification of medical protocols was the easiest issue to arrange. Stakeholders attended bilateral meetings to learn how the two systems worked and French and Catalan counterparts agreed on the medical equipment needed at Cerdanya Hospital. In general differences in protocols were rapidly resolved using scientific criteria, resulting in the following areas of agreement (Interview 2).

Pharmaceuticals

The French health system permits the use of drugs outside the international drug consensus, according to interviewees (Interviews 2 and 3). The solution is for the new hospital to use generic products under Spanish law.

Services and protocols

Several in-depth discussions took place on how to manage within Cerdanya Hospital certain treatments or services currently practised differently on each side of the border. Significant differences in treatment occur in the field of nephrology, for example, as French doctors use autodialysis with some patients while in Catalonia haemodialysis is more common (this solution is still under discussion). Actors agreed to use Catalan protocols for obstetrics as these tend to follow the patient more intensively, and decided to use French protocols for radiology services as these are more exigent than the Catalan equivalent. Where a medical service is only available on one side of the border, as in the case of orthopaedic surgery, the solution agreed is to follow the protocols of the country providing the service. The ultimate objective is that Cerdanya Hospital will offer a full array of health care services as provided by both the French and the Catalan health care systems.

---

6   Regulation (EEC) No 1612/68 of the Council of 15 October 1968 on freedom of movement for workers within the Community. *Official Journal of the European Union*, L 257: 2–12 (http://eur-lex.europa.eu/LexUriServ/ LexUriServ.do?uri=DD:I:1968_II:31968R1612:EN:PDF, accessed 9 July 2013).

Primary care

As noted earlier different systems exist in each country. The French health care system uses a model based on private family doctors who follow up with patients throughout their lives. In Catalonia family doctors working in primary health care centres and multidisciplinary teams tend to act as gatekeepers, referring patients to specialists. In this particular case, the aim is to achieve equilibrium on a win–win basis so that no parties feel they are losing "their" patients. The hope is that French doctors will refer patients to Cerdanya Hospital instead of Perpignan.

Clinical records

These are very similar in both countries and are unlikely to give rise to problems. In fact, the new hospital plans to connect the Catalan and the French system of clinical histories. The remaining outstanding question concerns how to protect the data.

Administration and management

The first and most important issue in this category relates to merging "two cultures, two administrations and two countries with different political agendas" (Interview 4). The obstacles represented by the continual political changes in both countries clearly reflect this difficulty. In the last two decades there have been more than 30 elections in the territory, leading to several changes in the personnel of the administrations involved in the collaboration. They have resulted, for example, in three different mayors in Puigcerdà, four different governments in Catalonia and three in France, quite apart from internal changes within the French health care administration leading to the transformation of the regional hospital agency into several regional health agencies. These frequent changes in political agenda are, in the opinion of most stakeholders, the reason the hospital has postponed its opening so often. Adoption of the EGTC legal formula has partly dissociated Cerdanya Hospital from this problem, as it has gained a certain amount of autonomy to work independently from the administrative and political changes in each country.

Another example relates to the issue of purchasing – of medical equipment, for example. In principle, since the hospital is located in Catalan territory, such acquisitions should take place within the framework of local public law and through the centralized department of the Catalan Health Ministry. Instead of following this procedure, however, out of respect for the French collaboration partners the hospital management decided to use a more complex legal option consisting of calling for open tenders, thereby allowing French companies to bid for equipment supply contracts. Similarly, the design of new information technology for the hospital not only had to work with three languages but also needed to provide specific accounting information according to both Spanish and French laws. For this reason the hospital's investment in information systems represents a third of the total investment in equipment (Interview 4).

Other minor problems will also emerge as the stakeholders gain inaugural experience of the day-to-day operation of a cross-border care facility. These will be important and varied and may include issues such as the repatriation of deceased French patients' bodies and concerns surrounding people sent to the hospital under police arrest (since the French gendarmerie cannot carry weapons in Spanish territory). A Spanish or French doctor's decision to disqualify a patient on the grounds of mental health may not be recognized by their juridical counterpart, and even small details such as how to deal with ambulances that display different warning lights need to be addressed. Admittedly, none of these issues is entirely unforeseen, but different stakeholders perceived these specific problems as insurmountable obstacles during the course of the project and addressed them regularly in interviews.

Actors are, nevertheless, continually finding solutions to problems seen as insuperable even less than a year earlier. For instance, the issue of the nationality of French babies born at Cerdanya Hospital (in Catalonia) was partially solved by opening an office specifically to deal with the juridical process associated with neonates while a new law was approved (Renyé, 2011; Assemblée Nationale, 2011). (Deliveries by French women in Puigcerdà Hospital were not historically a problem because of the low numbers affected.)

One problem still under discussion is co-payments. While in France there is a broad system of co-payments, in Spain these are mainly restricted to certain prescribed medicines, so should Cerdanya Hospital apply them only to French patients and not Spanish ones? The floating population exacerbates this issue (BOE, 2011): if the hospital applies co-payments only to patients from France does this give rise to a discriminatory issue?

In summary, however, it is clear that stakeholders on both sides of the border have created initiatives to ensure the continuation of the project, overcoming the obstacles and solving the problems as they arise.

Conclusion

Two distinct periods are discernible in the development of the Cerdanya cross-border hospital. In the beginning local administrations took the joint initiative to build a new hospital as they could not meet their evolving health service requirements independently. Patients in Upper Cerdanya needed faster access to hospital services because of the difficult journey to the nearest French hospital in some conditions. Catalan Cerdanya needed new health facilities but its administration did not deem the investment worthwhile because of the scarcity of population during much of the year. At the same time the Catalan administration was seeking an opportunity to expand activities with higher added value and better-quality jobs. The history of cooperation between the two sides of the Cerdanya region undoubtedly facilitated the idea of constructing a cross-border hospital.

The second phase of the project began after the feasibility study of 2003, once it received approval from national and regional institutions. Administrations on both sides of the border included the hospital in territorial plans that sought to consolidate deeper changes within the region. Other cross-border initiatives such as the paediatric and geriatric health centres, a cross-border slaughterhouse, a water purification plant, and initiatives on higher education reinforced these changes, although many of them remain at the planning stage.

After 2004 when the project began to take shape and national and regional institutions became involved, local organizations progressively lost control over it. A side-effect of this was that once the larger administrations took over the project slowed down as a result of continual changes associated with the electoral cycle. In this phase the project faced multiple obstacles associated with adapting the different medical protocols, administrative laws and managerial systems or regulations to which both administrations are subject. Surprisingly, the differences in medical protocols were, relatively, the easiest to solve. Above all, it became clear that patients were the crucial element of the project and that the hospital's sustainability would depend on its ability to attract French patients and to respect the internal equilibrium of the health systems on each side of the border. The new hospital will need the support of all relevant stakeholders.

Building the cross-border hospital means that key groups of actors with little previous interaction will suddenly have to start cooperating closely, developing new roles and relationships; these changes are not always easy to accept, not least in a context where the health care sector is an important employer on both sides of the border. In Catalonia, the existing Puigcerdà Hospital Foundation will shift its activity to the new EGTC Cerdanya Hospital and Puigcerdà City Council, which for years had an important role in co-managing the old hospital, will transfer significant powers to the Catalan Health Service and Languedoc-Roussillon Regional Health Agency. In the words of one interviewee, the new hospital may be local, but its management has moved hundreds of kilometres away. On the French side recovery centres, currently struggling with underutilization, will need to convert their activities to support the new geriatric and paediatric health centres that will serve the whole region. To become truly cross-border the new hospital will have to appeal to local French patients, who are accustomed to choosing their health care providers freely. It thus plans to recruit both Catalan and French staff; this has the added benefit of absorbing personnel who may be made redundant by the rationalization of older recovery centres. French family doctors will also have to deal with a new context that could reduce their activity levels. Cerdanya Hospital has to gain their confidence and avoid any competition, not least because they will be instrumental in referring the French patients it needs to avoid making a financial loss. Creating a cross-border hospital is thus an ambitious, long-term project which extends far beyond the building of a new facility.

This study contributes to the existing literature on cross-border care experiences in Europe. The authors believe that one of the most important policy implications derived from the evidence is that the cross-border hospital has ushered in a new stage of political relationships based on mutual trust across the border, mainly between the regional administrations (see Figs. 9.1 and 9.2). The border is, nevertheless, a permanent fixture in the minds of many people in the region: even though the European process of political and economic integration has led to convergence between the two communities, they are still separate and distinct entities with their own rules, institutions and logic. Differences between the two health systems also reinforce the border.

The significant financial role played by the European Union (EU) was decisive for the project as without the ERDF funds it would not have got off the ground, but the EU had no involvement in either managing or helping to solve the political and legal problems that arose. European institutions could develop clearer leadership, providing legislative and political instruments in order to facilitate the implementation of cross-border care facilities. A roadmap and clear EU leadership could have avoided two major problems faced by the new hospital: the continual change of actors resulting from political elections and the lack of a clear vision of the final administrative, legal and managerial structure of the hospital.

Acknowledgements

The authors wish to thank Dr Jordi Boix, Dr Franzina Riu and Dr Enric Subirats (Puigcerdà Hospital), Dr Felip Benavent (Pyrenees Health Region), Dr Xavier Conill (Calella Hospital), Mr Albert Piñeira (Mayor of Puigcerdà), Mr Jean-Jacques Fortuny (Mayor of Bourg-Madame), Mr Joan Planella (former Mayor of Puigcerdà), Ms Rose de Montellà, Mr Jacques Arevalo (Association Joseph Sauvy) and Mr Ricard Bellera (CCOO Trade Union) for providing the core information for this study via interview. The authors extend their gratitude to Ms Maria Cano (Puigcerdà Hospital) for her valuable help.

References

Actualitat La Cerdanya (2012). L'hospital transfronterer obrirà d'aquí 1 any [The cross-border hospital opens in 1 year] [web site]. Puigcerdà, Pirineus TV (www.pirineustelevisio.com/2012/06/hospital-transfronterer-obrira-en-un-any/, accessed 8 July 2013).

Assemblée Nationale (2011). *Proposition de Loi No. 3485 visant à permettre aux officiers de l'état civil français d'enregistrer les déclarations de naissance au sein de l'hôpital transfrontalier commun à la France et à l'Espagne.* Paris, Assemblée Nationale (www.assemblee-nationale.fr/13/propositions/pion3485.asp, accessed 9 July 2013).

BOE (2011). Resolución de 13 de diciembre de 2010, de la Secretaría General Técnica, por la que se publica la inscripción de los estatutos de la "Agrupación Europea de Cooperación Territorial Hospital de la Cerdaña" [Resolution of December 13, 2010, of the Technical Secretariat, on publishing the registration of the statutes of the "European Grouping of Territorial Cooperation Hospital de la Cerdanya"]. *Boletin Oficial del Estado,* 36, 11-2-11, Sec. III: 14875–94.

Boix J (2011). EU Territorial Health Care Project of Cerdanya. Projet Européen de Santé de Territoire de Cerdagne. [presentation]. *ECAB (Evaluating Care Across Borders) Project, Second Meeting, Universitat de Barcelona,17–18 January 2011.*

Bourret C, Tort i Bardolet J (2003). Maîtrise de l'information, amélioration des systèmes de santé et aménagement du territoire. L'exemple de la Catalogne (Espagne) et de la région Midi-Pyrénées. *International Journal of Info & Com Sciences for Decision-making*, 1: 162–72.

European Commission (2011). *Report from the Commission to the European Parliament and the Council. The application of the Regulation (EC) No 1082/2006 on a European Grouping of Territorial Cooperation (EGTC).COM(2011) 462 final.* Brussels, European Commission (www.interact-eu.net/downloads/4439/Commission_report_Application_of_the_EGTC_07_2011.pdf, accessed 5 July 2013).

Fundació Privada Hospital de Puigcerdà (2010). *Memòria 2009.* Puigcerdà, Fundació Privada Hospital de Puigcerdà (www.hospitalpuigcerda.com/pdf/menoria2009.pdf, accessed 8 July 2013).

Glinos IA, Baeten R (2006). *A literature review of cross-border patient mobility in the European Union.* Brussels, Observatoire social européen (www.ose.be/files/publication/health/WP12_lit_review_final.pdf, accessed 4 July 2013).

Harant P (2006). Hospital cooperation across French borders. In: Rosenmöller M, McKee M, Baeten R, eds. *Patient mobility in the European Union: learning from experience.* Copenhagen, WHO Regional Office for Europe: 157–77 (www.euro.who.int/__data/assets/pdf_file/0005/98420/ Patient_Mobility.pdf, accessed 4 July 2013).

Idescat (2010). The municipality in figures. Bank of statistics on municipalities and counties [web site]. Barcelona, Idescat (www.idescat.cat, accessed 10 September 2013).

Nys H, Goffin T (2011). Mapping national practices and strategies relating to patients' rights. In: Wismar M, Palm W, Figueras J, Ernst K and Van Ginneken E, eds. *Cross-border health care in the European Union: mapping and analysing practices and policies.* Copenhagen, WHO Regional Office for Europe on behalf of the European Observatory on Health Systems and Policies (Observatory Studies Series, No. 22: 159–216; www.euro.who.int/__ data/assets/pdf_file/0004/135994/e94875.pdf, accessed 9 July 2013).

POCTEFA (2008). Programa Operativo de Cooperación Territorial España-Francia-Andorra [Spain-France-Andorra Territorial Operative Cooperation Programme] [web site]. Jaca, POCTEFA (www.poctefa.eu/, accessed 5 July 2013).

Renyé A (2011). L'hospital no serà transfronterer per als nadons i els morts de l'Alta Cerdanya [The hospital will not be a cross-border hospital for babies and deceased people of Upper Cerdanya], El Punt, 11 March (www.elpuntavui.cat/noticia/article/1-territori/12-infraestructures/ 380225-lhospital-no-sera-transfronterer-per-als-nadons-i-els-morts-de-lalta-cerdanya.html, accessed 9 July 2013).

Rodríguez C, Conill X (2003). *Project Interreg iiia final report: Estudi de Viabilitat pel Desenvolupament d'un Hospital Comú Transfronterer a la Cerdanya (Baixa i Alta Cerdanya i el Capcir) [Viability study for the development of a common cross-border hospital in the Cerdanya (Lower and Upper Cerdanya and Capcir)].* Barcelona, CHC Consultoria i Gestió, SA.

Salvat M, Vigo M, Macbeth H, Bertranpetit J (1997). Seasonality of marriages in Spanish and French parishes in the Cerdanya valley, eastern Pyrenees. *Journal of Biosocial Science,* 29(1): 51–62.

Tobar Pascual C (2003). Sanitary cross-border cooperation: reality or fiction? The experience in la Cerdanya. In: *Free movement and cross-border cooperation in Europe: the role of hospitals and practical experiences in hospitals, proceedings of the HOPE Conference and Workshop, Luxembourg, June 2003.* Luxembourg, Entente des hôpitaux luxembourgeois.

Annex 9.1 Interviews conducted

Number	Date	Interviewee	Institution
Interview 1	4 May 2011; 7 June 2011	Dr Jordi Boix, General Manager; member of the board of directors of EGTC Cerdanya Hospital	Puigcerdà Hospital
Interview 2	25 November 2011	Dr Franzina Riu, Medical Director and Dr Enric Subirats, Head of Internal Medicine	Puigcerdà Hospital
Interview 3	6 September 2011	Dr Xavier Conill, Co-author of the viability study	Calella Hospital
Interview 4	3 November 2011	Dr Felip Benavent, Operations Director of the Pyrenees Health Region; member of the board of directors of EGTC Cerdanya Hospital	Catalan Health Service
Interview 5	23 September 2011	Ms Rose de Montellà, President of Association Joseph Sauvy; member of the consultative body of EGTC Cerdanya Hospital	Joseph Sauvy Centre
Interview 6	23 September 2011	Mr Jacques Arevalo, Director of Association Joseph Sauvy	Joseph Sauvy Centre
Interview 7	30 September 2011	Mr Albert Piñeira, current Mayor of Puigcerdà; Secretary of the Puigcerdà Hospital Foundation; member of the consultative body of EGTC Cerdanya Hospital	Puigcerdà City Council
Interview 8	16 September 2011	Mr Joan Planella, former secretary of Puigcerdà Hospital; former Alderman and Mayor of Puigcerdà 2007–2011	Puigcerdà City Council
Interview 9	30 September 2011	Mr Jean-Jacques Fortuny, Mayor of Bourg-Madame 1995–2011; member of the consultative body of EGTC Cerdanya Hospital	Bourg-Madame City Council
Interview 10	14 June 2011	Mr Ricard Bellera, Responsible for the international policy of the Catalan section of CCOO Trade Union	CCOO – Catalan section

Annex 9.2 French recovery centres in Upper Cerdanya, 2003

Name	Age group treated	Private/ public	Type of recovery	Location	Beds
Clinique du Souffle la Solane	Adults	Private	Chronic respiratory illness	Osséja	68
Le Soleil Cerdan	Adults	Private	Pneumology and recovery	Osséja	80
Charles et Madona	Adults	Private	Psychiatric recovery	Osséja	60
Val Pyrène	Adults	Private	Alcohol and drug recovery	Odeillo	52
Centre des Escaldes	Adults	Public	Respiratory and polyvalent recovery	Les Escaldes	150
Via sol	Children	Private	MECSS	Font Romeu	40
Castel Roc	Children	Private	MECSS	Font Romeu	40
Les Ailes d'Éole	Children	Private	MECSS	Font Romeu	40
Les Petits Lutins	Children	Private	MECSS	Font Romeu	40
Le Nid Soleil	Children	Private	MECSS	Font Romeu	40
Le Mas Catalan	Children	Private	MECSS	Font Romeu	40
Les Touts Petits	Children	Private	MECSS	Bourg-Madame	40
La Perle Cerdane	Children	Public	MECSS	Bourg-Madame	115
Joseph Sauvy Centre	All ages	Private	Rural Clinic	Err	22
Total					**827**

Source: Rodríguez and Conill, 2003.
Note: MECSS stands for Maison d'Enfants à Caractère Sanitaire et Social.